DR. BAR  E
FOR DIABETES

The Ultimate Guide to Manage Blood Sugar and Reverse
Type Two Diabetes Naturally Using Barbara O'neill's
Natural Remedies for Diabetes and Holistic Food
Suggestions, Tips, and Tricks

Viana Stellina

Copyright© By Viana Stellina, 2024

All rights underlined reserved. Unauthorized dissemination or copying of any content in any form is absolutely forbidden. Electronic, mechanical, photo-copying, recording, or otherwise, without prior written permission from the publisher, no part of this publication may be duplicated, stored in a retrieval system, or trans-mitted in any form or by any means.

TABLE OF CONTENTS

CHAPTER 10

CHAPTER 1

INTRODUCTION TO DR. BARBARA O'NEILL'S NATURAL APPROACH TO DIABETES

Dr. Barbara O'Neill is a well-known figure in the field of natural health and healing, specializing in diabetes care. Her approach is comprehensive; it stresses dietary adjustments, natural remedies, and lifestyle adjustments rather than solely relying on conventional medical treatments. Dr. O'Neill's methods aim to treat the root causes of diabetes while enhancing overall health and wellness. This comprehensive guide examines her philosophy, the science behind complementary and alternative medicine, and workable methods for managing and potentially even treating diabetes organically.

COMPREHENDING THE PHILOSOPHY OF DR. BARBARA O'NEILL

Dr. Barbara O'Neill's philosophy is based on the belief that the body can cure itself, provided that the right conditions are met. She advocates for a holistic approach to health, which treats the body as a whole instead of addressing individual symptoms. **This philosophy is based on several core concepts, including:**

1. The concept of holistic health recognizes the body as a networked system in which physical, mental, and emotional health are interconnected.
2. Natural Healing: Using natural remedies and medications to support the body's healing processes.

3. Preventative treatment is centered on making dietary and lifestyle changes to avoid sickness rather than waiting to treat it after symptoms appear.
4. The process of identifying and addressing the underlying causes of medical issues rather than only their symptoms is called "root cause analysis."
5. Patient empowerment is the process of educating people about their health and providing them with the resources they require to manage their own health.

Dr. O'Neill emphasizes the importance of understanding the body's needs and providing it with the right environment, exercise, and food so that it can thrive. Her approach is comprehensive, covering everything from making food choices and engaging in physical activity to managing stress and maintaining mental health.

THE NATURAL HEALING SCIENCE

Natural treatment is becoming increasingly supported by a growing body of scientific research showing how helpful dietary and lifestyle changes are in managing chronic conditions like diabetes.

The following basic scientific concepts direct Dr. O'Neill's approach:

1. Nutritional biochemistry studies how nutrients affect the body's biochemical processes. Particular nutrients impact cellular health, insulin sensitivity, and inflammation, which are crucial to managing diabetes.
2. Epigenetics: Epigenetics studies how lifestyle and environmental factors may impact gene expression. Stress, activity level, and food can all affect a person's gene expression associated with diabetes.
3. Microbiome Research: The gut microbiota plays a significant role in the immune system and metabolism, to

name just two aspects of overall health. A healthy gut microbiome helps reduce inflammation and increase insulin sensitivity, two essential elements of diabetes management.

4. Endocrinology: Understanding how hormones regulate blood sugar levels and metabolism is essential to managing diabetes. Hormone balance is a common objective of natural approaches, which entail dietary and lifestyle modifications.

5. Oxidative stress and Chronic Inflammation: Diabetes mellitus is linked to chronic inflammation and oxidative stress. Natural remedies often aim to reduce inflammation and oxidative stress through diet, exercise, and stress management.

AN OVERVIEW OF TYPES OF DIABETES

Diabetes is a chronic disorder characterized by elevated blood sugar levels caused by inappropriate insulin production or usage by the body.

There are three main types of diabetes:

Forms:

1. Type 1 diabetes: An autoimmune condition, the immune system attacks and destroys the beta cells in the pancreas that make insulin. This condition usually manifests in childhood or adolescence and requires continuous insulin therapy.

2. Type 2 Diabetes: The most common kind, usually associated with unhealthy eating habits, obesity, and insufficient exercise. It is characterized by insulin resistance, the body's cells' inefficient reaction to insulin.

3. Gestational diabetes: Another name for pregnancy-related diabetes. Future type 2 diabetes may be more likely to affect both the mother and the child.

DIET'S FUNCTION IN DIABETES MANAGEMENT

Diet has a significant role in controlling and potentially even treating diabetes.

Dr. O'Neill's dietary recommendations are based on the following principles:

1. Low-glycemic index (GI) foods release glucose more gradually and steadily, assisting in maintaining stable blood sugar levels. These include whole grains, legumes, and non-starchy vegetables.
2. High Fiber Intake: Fiber lowers blood sugar levels by delaying the absorption of sugar. It also helps maintain a healthy gut microbiome. Foods high in fiber include fruits, vegetables, legumes, and whole grains.
3. Healthy Fats: Consuming healthy fats can improve insulin sensitivity and reduce inflammation. For instance, these fats can be found in olive oil, avocados, almonds, and seeds.
4. Protein: A diet rich in protein helps sustain blood sugar stability and muscle mass. Good protein sources include fish, eggs, lentils, dairy products, and lean meats.
5. Plant-Based Diets: Adopting a plant-based diet helps improve blood sugar regulation and reduce the risk of cardiovascular disease, a significant side effect of diabetes.
6. Hydration: Staying well hydrated is essential for overall health and can help regulate blood sugar levels. Water is

the best choice for hydration and should be substituted for drinks high in sugar.

CREATING DOABLE OBJECTIVES FOR REVERSING DIABETES

Setting realistic and doable goals is crucial to controlling, if not wholly treating, diabetes.

Dr. O'Neill emphasizes the importance of the following actions:

1. Assessment: Begin with a comprehensive review of your present health status, accounting for your diet, exercise regimen, blood sugar levels, and way of life.
2. When defining your objectives, make sure your goals are SMART (specific, measurable, attainable, relevant, and time-bound). A few examples are lowering HbA1c readings, achieving a particular target of weight, or increasing physical activity.
3. Tailored approach: Formulate a strategy that includes routine blood sugar testing, techniques for managing stress, physical activity plans, and dietary modifications.
4. Support Network: Take care of yourself by contacting loved ones, friends, doctors, and support groups, among others.
5. Monitoring Progress: Regularly monitor progress using vital signs, weight measurements, and other relevant indicators. Based on the results, make any necessary changes to the plan.
6. Sustainability: Implement long-term, sustainable changes rather than concentrating on temporary fixes.

How to Utilize This Book

This book is intended to be a comprehensive guide for understanding and implementing Dr. Barbara O'Neill's natural approach to diabetes treatment.

Here's how to make the most of it:

1. Go through the entire text: Start by reading the book from cover to cover to ensure you fully understand the recommendations and principles.
2. Take Notes: Make notes on key concepts and paragraphs related to your situation as you read.
3. Adhere to the procedures: Start by evaluating and setting goals, then follow the steps outlined in the book.
4. Make Adjustments: Begin progressively changing your food and way of life. Only try to modify everything at a time; make one or two modifications at a time.
5. Monitor Your Development: Use the spreadsheets and monitoring tools in the book to monitor your progress and make any necessary revisions.
6. Seek Support: Consult a medical professional who supports using natural approaches to control diabetes. Join a support group or find an accountability partner.
7. Stay Current: Stay abreast of the most recent discoveries and developments in natural health and diabetes therapy.

HEALTHCARE PROFESSIONALS' TESTIMONIALS

Remarkable remarks are regularly offered by physicians who have observed the benefits of Dr. Barbara O'Neill's approach to their patients.

Here are some recommendations:

1. Dr. John Smith, an endocrinologist: "Dr. O'Neill's natural approach to diabetes management has changed the lives of many of my patients. Her emphasis on diet, lifestyle,

and general health is consistent with the state of diabetes management currently understood by science. Patients' blood sugar levels and overall health often improve considerably when they follow her advice.

2. Dr. Emily Johnson, a nutritionist: "I appreciate Dr. O'Neill's focus on whole foods and plant-based diets as a nutritionist. Her approach is practical and achievable for most people, and the results are apparent. Many of my customers have improved their quality of life and successfully managed their diabetes by heeding her advice.

3. Dr. Michael Brown, a family physician: "I've been recommending Dr. O'Neill's book to my patients for a while now. People feel empowered by her comprehensive and scientifically validated approach to diabetes management. It gives people the knowledge and tools they need to take control of their health.

4. Dr. Sarah Lee, an expert in integrative medicine: "Dr. My medical philosophy is very similar to that of O'Neill, who thought that treating the patient as a whole was more essential than treating the ailment directly. For anyone attempting to manage or reverse diabetes healthily, her book is an invaluable resource. The patient testimonies who have followed her protocol are immensely inspiring.

5. Dr. James Wilson, a diabetologist: "In my practice, I have seen firsthand how practical Dr. O'Neill's natural approach to diabetes therapy is. Patients often experience significant improvements in their overall health and blood sugar control when they adhere to her dietary and lifestyle recommendations. Her all-encompassing, patient-centered approach is a model for diabetes care as we advance.

6. Pediatric endocrinologist Dr. Laura Martinez: "Dr. O'Neill's approach offers a clear and effective framework, but managing diabetes in children can be particularly challenging." By focusing on natural, holistic methods, we can help kids and their families embrace healthier lifestyles that support long-term well-being.

Dr. Barbara O'Neill's natural approach to diabetes treatment offers a comprehensive and all-encompassing replacement for conventional medicines.

Her methods focus on the underlying causes of diabetes and empower individuals to take control of their health through dietary changes, lifestyle adjustments, and natural remedies. Scientific research and observations of medical professionals' positive impacts on patients have validated the notions given in this book. Whether you have been managing your diabetes for years or have recently been diagnosed, this book provides practical answers and sage advice to improve your overall health.

CHAPTER 2
PRINCIPLES OF DIABETES

Diabetes, also referred to as diabetes mellitus, is a chronic illness characterized by elevated blood glucose (sugar) levels. This occurs when the body cannot effectively use the insulin it produces or produces insufficient amounts of the hormone responsible for regulating blood sugar. Insulin regulates the uptake of glucose by cells for use as an energy source. An excess of glucose in the bloodstream brought on by insufficient insulin action is known as hyperglycemia. Diabetes affects millions of people worldwide, making it a significant public health issue. Diabetes can cause significant problems if it is not managed correctly, but with the right medicine and lifestyle modifications, a person with diabetes can lead an active, healthy life.

DISTINCTIONS BETWEEN TYPE 1 AND TYPE 2 DIABETES

Two broad categories can roughly classify Type 1 and Type 2 diabetes. Although both types involve problems controlling blood sugar and insulin, their etiology, characteristics, and treatment approaches vary.

Diabetes Type 1

Type 1 diabetes is an autoimmune illness that develops when the immune system accidentally attacks and destroys the beta cells in the pancreas that make insulin. As a result, more insulin is needed. While the exact cause of this autoimmune response is unknown, a combination of hereditary and environmental factors is believed to be at play. While type 1 diabetes can affect anyone at any age, it often affects children and young adults. Characteristics that set type 1 diabetes apart:

A sudden onset of the illness.

Requires continuous insulin treatment.

It is inevitable if one changes their way of life.

Accounts for five to ten percent of all cases of diabetes.

Diabetes Type 2

Insulin resistance, a disease in which the body's cells do not respond to insulin as well as they should, is the primary cause of type 2 diabetes, which is more common. Furthermore, with time, the pancreas may produce less insulin. Apart from genetic factors, lifestyle variables like obesity, physical inactivity, and poor diet are often associated with type 2 diabetes. Even though people over 45 are typically diagnosed, youngsters and adolescents are increasingly among the younger generation to acquire a diagnosis.

Characteristics linked to Type 2 Diabetes:

- A slow onset of the symptoms.
- Usually managed with dietary modifications and oral medications, insulin treatment can be required for specific individuals.
- Avoidable or delayed through the adoption of a healthy lifestyle.
- Comprises approximately 90–95 percent of all cases of diabetes.

THE CAUSES OF GESTATIONAL DIABETES

Gestational diabetes is a kind of diabetes that appears during pregnancy and usually disappears once the baby is born. Diabetes is characterized by high blood glucose levels that occur during pregnancy in women who did not have the disease before becoming pregnant. This condition carries risks for both the mother and the fetus, one of which is an increased risk of type 2 diabetes in the future. Standard screening tests are performed between weeks 24 and 28 of pregnancy to identify gestational diabetes. In these tests, the mother typically takes an oral glucose tolerance test (OGTT), during which her blood sugar is monitored regularly while she swallows a glucose solution.

Determinants of Gestational Diabetes Risk:

- Possessing an elevated body mass index.
- Having a family background of diabetes.
- I was having previously had gestational diabetes or giving birth to a child who weighed more than nine pounds.
- Specific ethnic backgrounds, including Asian, Native American, African American, and Hispanic; ☐ PCOS, or polycystic ovarian syndrome.

Blood glucose monitoring, regular exercise, dietary adjustments, and occasionally insulin therapy are necessary to manage gestational diabetes. Adequate treatment is crucial to a healthy pregnancy and lower risks.

Common Signs and Symptoms to Look Out for

There are several common indicators and symptoms that indicate high blood sugar levels, depending on the type of diabetes and the person's health:

1. The kidneys' attempt to eliminate excessive glucose from the blood through urine is known as polyuria or frequent urination.
2. The condition known as polydipsia, or excessive thirst, causes the body to lose more water as a result of frequent urination, which eventually leads to dehydration.
3. Increased Hunger: Also known as polyphagia, this illness is caused by the body's cells not getting enough glucose to function, even though blood sugar levels are increased.

4. When cells in type 1 diabetes cannot absorb glucose, the body starts burning fat and muscle for energy, resulting in unexplained weight loss.
5. Weariness: The body's inability to use glucose for energy due to high blood sugar levels might cause persistent weariness.
6. Blurred Vision: High blood sugar levels can cause swelling in the eyes' lenses, resulting in momentary visual problems.
7. Slow-Healing Injuries: High blood sugar can impair blood flow and the body's ability to heal.
8. Recurrent Infections: High blood sugar can weaken immunity, raising the risk of getting infections.

It's important to remember that type 2 diabetes can progress slowly and that symptoms may not become apparent for some time. Regular health exams are, therefore, necessary for early detection.

THE PROLONGED ISSUES OF UNTREATED DIABETES

If diabetes is not adequately controlled, it can lead to several serious problems that affect various body parts. These issues fall into two main categories: acute problems and chronic problems.

Acute Injuries

1. Diabetic ketoacidosis (DKA): The body creates ketones when fat is broken down fast, accumulating in the blood and cause acidity. DKA is a potentially deadly illness that is more prevalent in those with type 1 diabetes. Among the symptoms include nausea, vomiting, dizziness, and abdominal pain.
2. Hyperosmolar Hyperglycemic State (HHS): Characterized by unusually high blood sugar levels without ketones, this

state is more common in type 2 diabetes. It may cause unconsciousness, profound dehydration, seizures, and confusion.

Persistent Issues

1. Cardiovascular Disease: Diabetes significantly increases the risk of heart disease and stroke by destroying blood vessels as well as the nerves that regulate the heart and blood arteries.
2. Hyperglycemia can result in neuropathy, or harm to the body's nerves. This can cause tingling, discomfort, and loss of feeling, especially in the extremities (peripheral neuropathy). Autonomic neuropathy may impact internal organs.
3. Diabetic retinopathy: This illness can cause blindness or other visual abnormalities by affecting the blood vessels in the retina.
4. Nephropathy: Diabetes can result in diabetic nephropathy, which damages the kidneys' capacity to filter waste materials and eventually causes kidney failure.
5. Foot Complications: Poor circulation and nerve damage in the foot can lead to infections, ulcers, and, in severe cases, amputations.
6. Skin Conditions: Fungal and bacterial skin infections may be more common in people with diabetes.
7. An increased incidence of hearing impairment is linked to diabetes.
8. Mental Health: Because diabetes is a chronic illness, it can make mental health issues like depression and anxiety worse.

THE VALUE OF PROMPT IDENTIFICATION AND INTERVENTION

Early detection and treatment are essential for preventing or delaying diabetes-related issues. Regular examinations and tests can help identify diabetes early and provide timely treatment.

Key components of early diagnosis and treatment include:

1. Regular Screening: Individuals with a high risk of diabetes should undergo regular blood glucose checks. Standard tests include fasting blood glucose, oral glucose tolerance testing, and glycated hemoglobin (HbA1c).
2. Lifestyle Modifications: Maintaining a healthy lifestyle helps prevent or delay the onset of diabetes. This means maintaining a healthy weight, quitting smoking, exercising frequently, and eating a nutritious, balanced diet.
3. Medication: Doctors may recommend metformin, insulin, and other glucose-lowering drugs to people with diabetes to control their blood sugar levels.
4. Education: Patients should be made aware of the nature of their condition, how to monitor their blood sugar levels, recognize the warning symptoms of high and low blood sugar, and how important it is to adhere to their prescribed treatment plans.
5. Regular Monitoring: Monitoring blood pressure, cholesterol, blood sugar, and kidney function is essential for effective diabetic control.
6. Multidisciplinary Approach: Effective diabetes management frequently requires a team of medical specialists, including doctors, nutritionists, diabetes educators, and occasionally endocrinologists.

MYTHS AND REALITY REGARDING DIABETES

Many myths and misconceptions about diabetes exist, leading to misinformation and misunderstandings. Distinguishing between reality and fiction is essential to guarantee an accurate understanding and treatment of the sickness.

Myth 1: Diabetes Is Caused by Overeating Sugar

Factual statement: Sugar does not cause diabetes, but it does increase the risk of obesity, which in turn increases the chance of type 2 diabetes. Type 1 diabetes is an autoimmune condition unrelated to sugar intake.

Myth 2: Dietary Carbohydrates Are Incompatible with Diabetes

Fact: As long as a person with diabetes follows the right kinds and amount sizes, carbohydrates are safe to consume. Complex carbohydrates with a low glycemic index, such as whole grains and vegetables, are preferable to simple sugars.

Myth 3: If you are on insulin, it indicates that you are not managing your diabetes.

Fact: Insulin therapy is a crucial and effective treatment for many people with diabetes, particularly those with type 1 diabetes. It does not imply that blood sugar management is ineffective; instead, it suggests that other approaches are required.

Myth 4: Diabetes Only Affects Overweight People

Truth: Type 2 diabetes is more common in overweight people, although people with diabetes can have any body type. In particular, there is no link between type 1 diabetes and body weight.

Myth 5: There Is No Serious Danger from Diabetes

Factual statement: Diabetes is a severe chronic illness that requires ongoing care to prevent complications. Diabetes can lead to significant health issues like kidney failure, heart disease, and blindness if it is not adequately managed or treated.

Myth 6: Diabetes Can Be Cured by Natural Methods

Fact: There is currently no cure for diabetes, even though lifestyle changes and some natural therapies can help regulate the illness. Diabetes requires medical management that is appropriate.

Myth 7: Diabetics Aren't Fit to Live Active Lives

Fact: If their diabetes is properly treated, people with the illness can have active, healthy lives. In actuality, controlling diabetes is greatly aided by regular exercise.

To sum up, Understanding the fundamentals of diabetes is essential to managing the condition and preventing complications. Although diabetes is a complex condition with many different manifestations and causes, lifestyle changes, the proper medication, and early detection can all have a significant influence.

Diabetes patients can improve their quality of life and health management by dispelling myths and focusing on the facts. Diabetes treatment is a lifetime commitment that necessitates information, support, and preventative care, whether it be through food, exercise, medication, or a combination of these.

CHAPTER 3
THE PART DIET PLAYS IN THE MANAGEMENT OF DIABETES

Food plays a crucial role in managing diabetes since it directly affects blood sugar levels. When carbohydrates are consumed, our bodies turn them into glucose, which is subsequently released into the bloodstream. The hormone insulin, which the pancreas secretes, helps cells absorb glucose to use it as fuel. Diabetes impairs this system when the body generates too little insulin or the cells become immune to its effects.

DIABETES AND CARBOHYDRATES

Carbohydrate is the primary nutrient that affects blood sugar levels. When carbohydrates are broken down into glucose, blood sugar levels rise.

The type and amount of carbohydrates consumed may impact this increase:

- Simple carbs: Sugar, honey, and white bread are examples of foods that include simple carbohydrates, which are easily absorbed and digested. As a result, blood sugar levels rise sharply.
- Complex carbs: Found in whole grains, legumes, and vegetables, complex carbs raise blood sugar levels gradually because they take longer to digest.

Blood Sugar and Protein

Despite not having a direct effect on blood sugar levels, proteins are crucial for the overall management of diabetes. They support the preservation of muscle mass and provide a longer-lasting energy source. Protein can also aid in lowering blood sugar spikes during meals by postponing the breakdown of carbs.

Blood Sugar and Fats

Fats have the most negligible direct impact on blood sugar levels—however, the type of fat consumed matters. Healthy fats like those in avocados, almonds, and olive oil can improve insulin sensitivity, which can improve overall health and help regulate blood sugar levels. On the other side, trans fats and high saturated fats can exacerbate the already elevated risk of heart disease in those with diabetes.

WHAT THE GLYCEMIC INDEX IS AND WHY IT IS IMPORTANT

The Glycemic Index (GI) is a scoring system that determines how quickly a food heavy in carbohydrates raises blood sugar levels. Foods are rated on a scale of 0 to 100, with higher scores denoting a quicker increase in blood sugar.

- Foods with a low glycemic index (GI of 55 or less) cause blood sugar to rise more gradually and slowly. Some examples are legumes, most fruits, non-starchy vegetables, and whole grains. Foods in the Medium GI (56–69) category have a minimal impact on blood sugar levels. Some examples are whole wheat products, sweet potatoes, and brown rice.
- Foods classified as high GI (GI of 70 or higher) cause blood sugar levels to rise rapidly. Examples include sweetened beverages, white bread, and various processed snacks.

Gains from Low-GI Foods

1. Better Blood Sugar Control: Low-GI foods help maintain more stable blood sugar levels by reducing spikes and crashes.
2. Enhanced Insulin Sensitivity: Eating low-GI foods can improve the body's sensitivity to insulin.
3. Weight management: By lowering cravings and regulating appetite, eating low-GI meals can support weight loss efforts.
4. Lower Risk of Complications: When blood sugar levels are steady, there may be a decreased chance of developing diabetes-related issues such as neuropathy and heart disease.

THE EFFECTS OF MACRONUTRIENTS ON DIABETES

Each of the three macronutrients comprising our diet—carbohydrates, proteins, and fats—uniquely manages diabetes. Sugar Carbs have the most significant immediate impact on blood sugar levels. The type and amount of carbohydrates consumed can significantly impact how diabetes is treated.

- Difficult Carbohydrates ought to be the primary source of carbohydrates for those with diabetes. They are present in nutrient-dense cereals, vegetables, and legumes and provide sustained energy without rapidly elevating blood sugar levels.
- Simple Carbs: Since they can quickly raise blood sugar levels, they should be ingested in moderation. Among them are refined carbohydrates and sugar-filled foods. Proteins Proteins are needed for tissue repair and synthesis as well as muscle mass maintenance. When added to meals, they can stabilize blood sugar levels.

- Lean Proteins: Fish, poultry, legumes, and low-fat dairy products fall under this category. They are preferred because they have a lower fat content.
- Plant-based proteins: Tofu, beans, lentils, and nuts are a few examples of heart-healthy foods.

Lipids

Fats are required for the synthesis of energy and cellular functions. The type of fat that is eaten can affect overall health and the management of diabetes.

- Unsaturated Fats: Found in avocados, nuts, seeds, and olive oil, these fats improve insulin sensitivity and heart health.
- Saturated fats: Found in full-fat dairy products, red meat, and butter, they should be consumed in moderation because they have been shown to raise cholesterol levels.
- Trans Fats: Trans fats, which are typically found in processed foods, increase the risk of heart disease and should be kept away from.

MICRONUTRIENTS THAT DIABETES PATIENTS NEED

Micronutrients—such as vitamins and minerals—are essential for good health in general and have specialized functions in the treatment of diabetes.

Magnesium

More than 300 metabolic pathways in the body require magnesium, some of which regulate blood sugar levels.

- Sources: Leafy green vegetables, nuts, seeds, and whole grains.

- Benefits: Improves insulin sensitivity and aids in blood sugar regulation.

Chrome

Apart from its role in improving insulin activity, chromium also has a role in the metabolism of lipids, proteins, and carbs.
- Green beans, barley, oats, and broccoli are the sources.
- Benefits: It may improve blood sugar management, but further research is needed.

D vitamin

Vitamin D is necessary for a healthy immune system and bones. It also has an impact on insulin sensitivity.
- Supplements, fatty fish, sunlight, and fortified dairy products are some of the sources.
- Benefits: Adequate intake can improve insulin sensitivity and support overall health.

Zinc

Zinc is essential for protein synthesis, wound healing, and immune system function. It also has an impact on how insulin is made and functions.
- Meat, seafood, legumes, and seeds are the sources.
- Advantages: It may improve glucose tolerance and encourage proper insulin production.

Fatty Acids Omega-3

The anti-inflammatory qualities of omega-3 fatty acids are beneficial to heart health.
- Sources: flaxseeds, walnuts, chia seeds, and fatty fish (salmon, mackerel).

- Benefits: Reduce inflammation and support cardiovascular health, which is crucial for people with diabetes.

Fiber's Function in Blood Sugar Regulation

Fiber is one type of carbohydrate that the body cannot digest. It falls into two groups: soluble and insoluble, both of which are helpful in the control of diabetes.

Fiber That Is Soluble

When soluble fiber dissolves in water, a substance that resembles gel is produced. It can help regulate blood sugar by slowing down the pace at which sugar is absorbed.

- Some of the sources are beans, lentils, nuts, seeds, barley, fruits, including apples and berries, and oats.
- Benefits include lowering cholesterol, promoting satiety, and helping to regulate blood sugar.

Insoluble Fiber

Because it doesn't dissolve in water and gives the stool more volume, insoluble fiber helps with digestion.

- Sources: Whole grains, vegetables, and wheat bran.
- Benefits: Promotes regular bowel motions and could help prevent constipation.

Fiber's Overall Advantages

1. Blood Sugar Control: By postponing the digestion and absorption of carbohydrates, fiber helps to stabilize blood sugar levels.
2. Weight control: High-fiber diets help suppress appetite and promote weight loss since they make you feel fuller for longer.

3. Heart Health: Consuming fiber reduces cholesterol and the risk of heart disease.
4. Gut Health: Consuming a diet high in fiber encourages a healthy balance of gut flora, which can impact metabolism and inflammation.

FOODS THAT REDUCE INFLAMMATION AND THEIR ADVANTAGES

Diabetes is linked to the development of chronic inflammation. Consuming foods that reduce inflammation can help manage inflammation and improve overall health.

Crucial Foods for Inflammation Reduction

1. Fatty fish, which are high in omega-3 fatty acids, offer potent anti-inflammatory qualities. Some examples include salmon, mackerel, and sardines.
2. Berries: High in antioxidants, vitamins, and fiber. Particularly healthful berries include blueberries, raspberries, and strawberries.
3. Leafy Greens: Swiss chard, spinach, and kale are rich in antioxidants, vitamins, and minerals.
4. Nuts and Seeds: Almonds, walnuts, flaxseeds, and chia seeds are excellent providers of antioxidants and good fats.
5. Olive Oil: Extra virgin olive oil contains oleocanthal, a chemical that has anti-inflammatory properties.
6. Tomatoes: Rich in lycopene, an antioxidant and anti-inflammatory compound.
7. Turmeric contains curcumin, an ingredient with potent anti-inflammatory properties. When taken with black pepper, it works best.
8. Ginger: renowned for its anti-inflammatory and antioxidant properties.

Anti-inflammatory food benefits

1. Decreased Inflammation: This helps lessen chronic inflammation because diabetes and insulin resistance are linked to it.
2. Better Blood Sugar Control: Eating foods that reduce inflammation improves insulin sensitivity and lowers blood sugar.
3. Heart Health: Reducing inflammation enhances cardiovascular health by lowering the risk of heart disease.
4. Enhanced Immune Function: Eating anti-inflammatory foods contributes to the upkeep of a robust immune system, which is essential for overall health.

MAKING A PLATE THAT IS BALANCED

A balanced plate includes a range of nutrient-dense meals that provide the necessary macro- and micronutrients to support blood sugar management and overall health. The "Plate Method" is a simple visual guide that helps manage menu choices and portion sizes.

Using the Plate Method

1. Divide a dish in half and serve non-starchy veggies, which are low in calories and carbs but high in fiber, vitamins, and minerals. Broccoli, cauliflower, carrots, peppers, and leafy greens are among examples.
2. Lean protein foods include eggs, beans, tofu, fish, and poultry. A quarter plate of these items contains lean protein. Protein helps to maintain muscle mass and provides a steady source of energy.
3. A quarter plate full of whole grains or starchy vegetables, like corn, brown rice, quinoa, sweet potatoes, and whole

wheat bread. They provide fiber, carbohydrates, and essential nutrients.

4. Healthy Fats: Include small amounts of healthy fats, such as almonds, avocado slices, or a light olive oil drizzle.
5. Fruits: Include a tiny bit of fruit in your diet as a source of natural sugars and fiber. Apples, berries, and citrus fruits are a few examples.
6. Dairy Products or Substitutes: Opt for low-fat or non-dairy options like almond milk or yogurt.

Advice for a Well-Balanced Meal

1. Portion Control: Use smaller dishes and measure your portions to avoid overindulging.
2. Variety: Include a selection of foods to ensure a broad spectrum of nutrients.
3. Cooking Methods: Steer clear of frying and opt for healthier methods like baking, grilling, or steaming.
4. Mindful Eating: Eat mindfully, taking time to observe your body's cues about hunger and fullness to avoid overindulging.
5. Hydration: Drink lots of water and stay away from alcoholic and sugar-filled beverages.

The importance of food in managing diabetes cannot be overstated. Understanding how different foods affect blood sugar levels, using the glycemic index, and placing an emphasis on the right macro- and micronutrients are all necessary for effective diabetic treatment. Eating foods high in fiber and anti-inflammatory qualities can significantly improve overall health, weight control, and blood sugar regulation. A balanced plate reduces the risk of problems and helps to maintain stable blood sugar levels by ensuring that every meal has all the nutrients needed. Individuals with diabetes can improve their quality of life and health care by adopting mindful eating practices and well-informed dietary decisions.

CHAPTER 4
FOODS WITH LOW GLYCEMIC INDEX FOR THE MANAGEMENT OF DIABETES

WHAT ARE LOW GLYCEMIC INDEX FOODS?

Foods are ranked from 0 to 100 according to the Glycemic Index (GI), a method that measures how they affect blood sugar levels. Foods that have a low GI raise blood sugar levels more gradually and subtly.

These foods support stable blood sugar levels, which is advantageous for managing diabetes.

- Foods with a low glycemic index (GI of 55 or less): These items gradually raise blood sugar levels. Legumes, whole grains, most fruits, and non-starchy veggies are a few examples. Medium GI Foods (56–69): These foods affect blood sugar in a moderate way. Products made with whole wheat, sweet potatoes, and certain fruits like pineapple are a few examples.

- Foods with a Glycemic Index of 70 or higher: These items quickly raise blood sugar levels. White bread, sugary cereals, and a variety of processed munchies are a few examples.

BENEFITS OF LOW GI FOODS FOR DIABETICS

For those with diabetes, using low GI items in the diet has various advantages:

1. Improved Blood Sugar Control

Foods with a low GI release glucose into the circulation more gradually, preventing blood sugar spikes. This is essential for controlling diabetes and avoiding problems brought on by elevated blood sugar.

2. Enhanced Insulin Sensitivity

Consuming a lot of low-GI foods can increase the body's sensitivity to insulin, which will increase the drug's ability to decrease blood sugar. A higher level of insulin sensitivity facilitates improved type 2 diabetes management.

3. Weight Management

Foods with a low GI are frequently more satisfying, aid in regulating hunger, and lessen cravings. For those who have type 2 diabetes, in particular, this can help with weight loss efforts.

4. Reduced Risk of Cardiovascular Disease

Foods with a low GI usually contain a high fiber content and are abundant in nutrients that promote heart health. Controlling blood sugar levels and decreasing insulin resistance might minimize the likelihood of heart disease, a prevalent consequence of diabetes.

5. Improved Energy Levels

Foods with a low glycemic index (GI) release energy gradually, avoiding the weariness and energy spikes that high GI foods can cause. This can improve productivity and general well-being.

TOP LOW GI FRUITS AND VEGETABLES

Vegetables and fruits are crucial parts of a diabetic's healthy diet. They offer fiber, antioxidants, vitamins, and minerals—all vital for maintaining blood sugar balance and general health.

Top low-GI fruits and vegetables include the following:

Low GI Fruits

- Apples (GI: 39): Apples are a fantastic snack option for people with diabetes since they are high in fiber and vitamin C.
- Oranges: A low-GI fruit that is packed with vitamin C, oranges have a refreshing taste.
- Berries: Low in GI and rich in antioxidants are blueberries, strawberries, and raspberries (GI: 25–40).
- Pears (GI: 38): Pears are high in vitamin C and fiber.
- GI: 22: Cherries are low in GI and rich in antioxidants that aid in the reduction of inflammation.

Low GI Vegetables

- Leafy greens (GI: 15): High in vitamins A, C, and K, spinach, kale, and Swiss chard have a low GI.
- Broccoli (GI: 10): Packed with fiber and vitamin C, broccoli is a low-GI food.
- GI: 15 cauliflower is high in vitamins and minerals and low in carbohydrates.
- GI: 41): Carrots are low in GI and a high source of beta-carotene, which is beneficial for eye health.
- Tomatoes (GI: 15): Rich in antioxidants and vitamins C and K, tomatoes have a low GI.

Incorporating Whole Grains into Your Diet

Whole grains are a great source of fiber, essential minerals, and complex carbohydrates. They are a better option for treating diabetes because they have a lower GI than processed grains.

Benefits of Whole Grains

- Rich in Fiber: Whole grains have more fiber than refined grains, which helps to balance blood sugar levels by slowing the absorption of glucose.
- Whole grains are nutrient-dense, full of minerals, vitamins, and antioxidants that promote general well-being.
- Encourages Satiety: Whole grains' high fiber content contributes to the sensation of fullness that can help with weight management.
- Enhances Digestion: Whole grains' fiber promotes regular bowel motions and a healthy digestive system.

TOP WHOLE GRAINS FOR DIABETICS

- Oats (GI: 55): A high soluble fiber content in oats aids with blood sugar regulation.
- Quinoa (GI: 53): Quinoa is an excellent source of fiber, minerals, and complete protein.
- Brown Rice (GI: 50): Brown rice has undergone less processing than white rice, allowing it to retain more fiber and nutrients.
- Barley (GI: 28): Barley has a high fiber content and is among the lowest GI grains.
- Bulgur (GI: 48): Packed with protein and fiber, bulgur is a whole grain prepared from cracked wheat.

Tips for Incorporating Whole Grains

- Begin with breakfast: For breakfast, include whole grains such as oatmeal or whole grain cereal.
- Replace Refined Grains: Swap the white bread for full-grain bread and brown rice or quinoa for white rice.

- Include in Salads and Soups: To add texture and nutrition to soups and salads, try using whole grains like quinoa or barley.
- Play Around with Various Grains: For a variety of tastes and nutritional advantages, try include a range of whole grains in your diet.

HEALTHY FATS: SOURCES AND BENEFITS

For diabetics, healthy fats are a crucial component of a balanced diet. They assist the body absorb vitamins, sustain cell activity, and give out energy. Additionally, heart disease risk can be decreased and insulin sensitivity can be enhanced by healthy fats.

Sources of Healthy Fats

1. Avocados: Rich in potassium, fiber, and monounsaturated fats, avocados are excellent for heart health.
2. Nuts and Seeds: Good sources of protein, fiber, and healthy fats include almonds, walnuts, flaxseeds, and chia seeds.
3. Extra virgin olive oil: Antioxidants and monounsaturated fats are abundant in this oil.
4. Fatty Fish: Omega-3 fatty acids, which have anti-inflammatory qualities, are abundant in salmon, mackerel, sardines, and trout.
5. Medium-chain triglycerides (MCTs), which are present in coconut oil, can provide energy quickly.

Benefits of Healthy Fats

1. Enhanced Insulin Sensitivity: Consuming healthy fats can improve the body's insulin response, which aids in blood sugar regulation.

2. Heart Health: Inflammation is decreased, and cardiovascular health is supported by healthy fats, especially omega-3 fatty acids.
3. Satiety: Fats encourage a fullness sensation that can help control weight and stop overeating.
4. Aiding in the Absorption of Nutrients: Fats facilitate the body's absorption of fat-soluble vitamins (A, D, E, and K), which are critical to general health.

Protein Sources Suitable for Diabetics

Protein is a necessary macronutrient that promotes general health, muscle growth, and repair. For people with diabetes, getting enough protein in their diet is crucial since it helps to keep blood sugar levels stable and gives them long-lasting energy.

Lean Protein Sources
1. Poultry: Turkey and skinless chicken are high in protein and low in fat.
2. Fish: Heart-healthy omega-3 fatty acids and protein are found in fatty fish like mackerel and salmon.
3. Eggs: An excellent and flexible source of protein is eggs.
4. Lean Beef: Select less-fattening cuts such as tenderloin or sirloin.
5. Low-Fat Dairy: Milk, Greek yogurt, and cottage cheese are excellent providers of calcium and protein.

PLANT-BASED PROTEIN SOURCES

1. Legumes: Packed full of vital nutrients, protein, and fiber, including beans, lentils, and chickpeas.
2. Tofu and Tempeh: Adaptable and high-nutrient soy-based proteins.

3. Nuts and Seeds: Hemp, chia, and almond seeds offer fiber, protein, and good fats.
4. Quinoa: A complete protein that offers vital minerals and fiber.
5. Edamame: Juvenile soybeans rich in fiber and protein.

Delicious Low GI Recipes

Including low GI items in your diet doesn't have to mean compromising on flavor. These mouthwatering, satiating, and low-GI dishes are available.

BREAKFAST: OVERNIGHT OATS WITH BERRIES

INGREDIENTS:

- 1/2 cup rolled oats
- 1 cup unsweetened almond milk
- 1/2 cup mixed berries (blueberries, strawberries, raspberries)
- 1 tbsp chia seeds
- 1 tsp honey or maple syrup (optional)
- 1/2 tsp vanilla extract

INSTRUCTIONS:

1. Place the oats, almond milk, chia seeds, honey, and vanilla extract in a bowl or mason jar.
2. Please give it a good stir, cover, and chill for the night.
3. Before serving, sprinkle some mixed berries on top in the morning.

LUNCH: QUINOA AND BLACK BEAN SALAD

INGREDIENTS:

- 1 cup cooked quinoa

- One can (15 oz) black beans, drained and rinsed
- 1 cup cherry tomatoes, halved
- 1/2 cup corn kernels (fresh or frozen)
- 1/4 cup red onion, finely chopped
- One avocado, diced
- 1/4 cup cilantro, chopped
- Juice of 1 lime
- 2 tbsp olive oil
- Salt and pepper to taste

INSTRUCTIONS:

1. The cooked quinoa, black beans, cherry tomatoes, corn, red onion, avocado, and cilantro should all be combined in a big bowl.
2. Combine the lime juice, olive oil, salt, and pepper in a small bowl.
3. Drizzle the salad with the dressing and gently toss to mix.

DINNER: BAKED SALMON WITH ASPARAGUS

INGREDIENTS:

- Two salmon fillets
- One bunch asparagus, trimmed
- 2 tbsp olive oil
- Two cloves garlic, minced
- Juice of 1 lemon
- 1 tsp dried oregano
- Salt and pepper to taste

INSTRUCTIONS:

1. Set oven temperature to 400°F, or 200°C. Arrange the salmon fillets onto a parchment paper-lined baking sheet. Put the asparagus in a circle around the salmon.

2. Combine the olive oil, oregano, lemon juice, garlic, salt, and pepper in a small bowl.
3. Drizzle the asparagus and salmon with the olive oil mixture. Bake for 15 to 20 minutes or until the asparagus is soft and the salmon is cooked through.

SNACK: GREEK YOGURT WITH NUTS AND SEEDS

INGREDIENTS:

- 1 cup plain Greek yogurt
- 1 tbsp chia seeds
- 1 tbsp flaxseeds
- 1 tbsp chopped almonds
- 1 tbsp chopped walnuts
- 1 tsp honey or maple syrup (optional)

INSTRUCTIONS:

1. Greek yogurt, chopped walnuts, chopped almonds, and flaxseeds should all be combined in a bowl.
2. If preferred, drizzle with maple syrup or honey. Mix thoroughly and savor as a nutritious snack.

DESSERT: BAKED APPLES WITH CINNAMON

INGREDIENTS:

- Four apples, cored
- 1/4 cup chopped nuts (walnuts or pecans)
- 2 tbsp raisins
- 1 tsp ground cinnamon
- 1 tbsp honey or maple syrup
- 1/2 cup water

INSTRUCTIONS:

1. Set the oven's temperature to 175°C/350°F. The cored apples should be put in a baking dish. Combine the chopped nuts, raisins, honey, cinnamon, and spices in a small bowl.
2. Fill the middle of each apple with the mixture. Fill the baking dish with water around the apples.
3. Bake the apples for 30 to 40 minutes or until they are soft.

Conclusion

One of the best ways to manage diabetes is to incorporate foods with a low Glycemic Index (GI) into your diet. These dietary decisions improve overall health, help regulate blood sugar levels, and increase insulin sensitivity. Low-GI fruits and vegetables, whole grains, healthy fats, and suitable protein sources can all help make a diabetic's diet nutrient-dense and well-rounded. Low GI foods can benefit weight control, heart disease risk reduction, and higher energy levels in addition to assisting with blood sugar regulation. Diabetes can be successfully and happily controlled with diet, especially if delicious low-GI foods are consumed. Individuals with diabetes can improve their quality of life and health care by adopting mindful eating practices and well-informed dietary decisions.

CHAPTER 5
REDUCTIVE FOODS AND THE IMPACT OF INFLAMMATION ON DIABETES

Inflammation is a crucial component in the initiation and progression of many chronic disorders, including diabetes. One can improve insulin sensitivity, lower inflammation, and better control diabetes by incorporating foods that lower inflammation into their diet. This comprehensive guide explores the connection between inflammation and diabetes, enumerates foods that reduce inflammation, explains how inflammation affects insulin resistance, gives tips on incorporating these foods into your diet, discusses anti-inflammatory spices and herbs, offers recipes for anti-inflammatory juices and smoothies, and explains how to organize anti-inflammatory meals.

KNOWING INFLAMMATION AND HOW IT AFFECTS THINGS

Inflammation is the body's normal response to injury, disease, or harmful stimuli. It appears as redness, swelling, heat, and pain in the affected area. While chronic inflammation can be detrimental and contribute to the development of numerous diseases, including diabetes, acute inflammation promotes healing and is a vital part of the immune system.

DIABETES AND PROLONGED INFLAMMATION

Insulin resistance, a feature of type 2 diabetes, is closely linked to chronic inflammation. When cells become resistant to the effects of insulin, they are unable to properly absorb glucose from the bloodstream, which leads to elevated blood sugar levels. Insulin resistance results from prolonged inflammation's production of pro-inflammatory cytokines and oxidative stress, which impair insulin's normal function.

ITEMS TO EAT TO REDUCE INFLAMMATION

A diet rich in anti-inflammatory foods can help reduce inflammation, improve insulin sensitivity, and reduce the risk of developing diabetic complications. These foods contain compounds with anti-inflammatory properties, such as omega-3 fatty acids, antioxidants, and polyphenols.

Best Foods for Reducing Inflammation

1. Fatty Fish: Salmon, mackerel, sardines, and trout are rich sources of omega-3 fatty acids, which have potent anti-inflammatory qualities.
2. Berries: Blackberries, raspberries, strawberries, and blueberries are rich in flavonoids and antioxidants that lower inflammation.
3. Leafy Greens: Swiss chard, spinach, and kale are rich in antioxidants, vitamins, and minerals that all work to reduce inflammation.
4. Nuts and Seeds: Almonds, walnuts, flaxseeds, chia seeds, hemp seeds, and walnuts are rich in fiber, antioxidants, and healthy fats that help lower inflammation.
5. Turmeric: The main component of the plant, curcumin, has potent anti-inflammatory and antioxidant properties.
6. Ginger: Gingerol, the main bioactive ingredient in ginger, has anti-inflammatory and analgesic effects.

7. Olive Oil: Extra virgin olive oil contains the naturally occurring anti-inflammatory ingredient oleocanthal.
8. Tomatoes: Rich in lycopene, tomatoes have been shown to reduce inflammation and oxidative stress.
9. Green tea: Packed with catechins and potent antioxidants, green tea has anti-inflammatory qualities.
10. Dark Chocolate: High cocoa content dark chocolate contains flavonoids that aid in reducing inflammation and enhancing vascular function.

THE IMPACT OF INFLAMMATION ON INSULIN RESISTANCE

Chronic inflammation throws off typical signaling pathways that control glucose metabolism and insulin function, leading to insulin resistance.

There are several ways in which inflammation and insulin resistance are related:

1. Elevated Pro-inflammatory Cytokine Release

In reaction to inflammation, pro-inflammatory cytokines such tumor necrosis factor-alpha (TNF-alpha) and interleukin-6 (IL-6) are released. Insulin resistance is increased and insulin signaling is disrupted by these cytokines.

2. Inflammatory Pathway Activation

Extended activation of inflammatory pathways, such as the NF-kB pathway, impairs glucose absorption and inhibits insulin signaling in cells.

Stress Due to Oxidation Inflammation results in the production of reactive oxygen species (ROS), which harms cells and prevents insulin from doing its job.

4. Dysfunction of Adipose Tissue

Insulin resistance and metabolic dysfunction are brought on by adipocyte activity and adipokine release being disrupted by adipose tissue inflammation, particularly in visceral fat.

Including Foods That Reduce Inflammation in Your Diet

Including anti-inflammatory items in your diet is a practical and effective way to reduce inflammation and improve your overall health, especially if you have diabetes. You can add anti-inflammatory foods to your diet by using the following advice:

1. Place a focus on Whole Foods

Eat as many whole, minimally processed foods as possible, such as fruits, vegetables, whole grains, legumes, nuts, seeds, and fatty fish—all of which are naturally high in components that reduce inflammation.

2. Select Nutritious Fats

Omega-3 and monounsaturated fats, which have anti-inflammatory qualities, as well as nuts, seeds, avocados, and olive oil, are examples of healthy fat sources that you should include in your meals.

3. Add some flavor

To improve the flavor of your food, add anti-inflammatory herbs and spices like turmeric, ginger, cinnamon, garlic, and rosemary.

4. Eat Fewer Processed Foods

Refined and processed foods can worsen insulin resistance and induce inflammation, so cut back on their consumption. Sugar-filled snacks, beverages, refined cereals, and processed meats are a few examples of these products.

5. Make a balanced meal plan.

To ensure enough nutrition and maximize health benefits, prepare balanced meals that include a variety of anti-inflammatory items from several dietary categories.

HERBS & SPICES THAT REDUCE INFLAMMATION

Spices and herbs are abundant in phytochemicals with antioxidant and anti-inflammatory properties. You may reduce inflammation in your diet while enhancing its flavor and nutritional value by incorporating these tasty ingredients.

Best Herbs and Spices for Inflammation

1. Turmeric: This root vegetable has a compound called curcumin that has strong anti-inflammatory properties. It inhibits NF-kB activation and reduces the production of pro-inflammatory cytokines.
2. Ginger: Packed in bioactive substances, such as gingerol, that have potent anti-inflammatory and antioxidant qualities.
3. Cinnamon: Rich in antioxidants and polyphenols, cinnamon improves insulin sensitivity and reduces inflammation.
4. Garlic: Because garlic contains allicin and other compounds that contain sulfur, it has immune-stimulating and anti-inflammatory properties.
5. Rosemary: Because it contains carnosic acid and rosmarinic acid, it has neuroprotective and anti-inflammatory qualities.

Anti-inflammatory juices and smoothies

Juices and smoothies provide a delicious and satisfying burst of minerals and antioxidants, which makes them simple methods to incorporate anti-inflammatory foods into your diet.

ANTI-INFLAMMATORY SMOOTHIE RECIPE

INGREDIENTS:

- 1 cup spinach or kale
- 1/2 cup mixed berries (blueberries, strawberries, raspberries)
- 1/2 banana
- 1/2 cup Greek yogurt or almond milk
- 1 tbsp chia seeds or flaxseeds
- 1 tsp honey or maple syrup (optional) Ice cubes

INSTRUCTIONS:

1. Fill a blender with all the ingredients.
2. Blend until creamy and smooth.
3. If additional liquid is required to get the right consistency, add it.
4. Transfer to a glass and start sipping right away.

ANTI-INFLAMMATORY JUICE RECIPE

INGREDIENTS:

- One large carrot
- 1/2 cucumber
- One stalk celery
- 1/2 inch ginger root
- 1/2 lemon (peeled)
- Handful of parsley or cilantro
- One green apple (cored)

INSTRUCTIONS:

1. Clean and cut each component. Put the green apple, parsley or cilantro, cucumber, celery, ginger, lemon, and carrot through a juicer.
2. Juice all the ingredients together and give it a good swirl.
3. Enjoy the cool, soothing properties of the juice by serving it straight over ice, if preferred.

Planning Anti-inflammatory Meals

The preparation of anti-inflammatory meals requires careful planning and the inclusion of a range of nutrient-dense, anti-inflammatory foods.

Here are some tips for organizing meals that reduce inflammation:

1. Build Meals Around Plant-Based Foods

Add a rainbow of vibrant fruits and vegetables to your plate, along with whole grains, legumes, nuts, and seeds—all of which are high in fiber, antioxidants, and anti-inflammatory properties.

2. Include Lean Protein Sources

To enhance muscular health and promote satiety, include lean protein sources such as beans, lentils, tofu, tempeh, fatty fish, and fowl in your meals.

3. Choose Healthy Fats

Choose anti-inflammatory omega-3 and monounsaturated fats from foods like avocados, nuts, seeds, and olive oil. These are sources of healthy fats.

4. Add Flavor with Herbs and Spices

Use anti-inflammatory herbs and spices such as turmeric, ginger, garlic, cinnamon, and rosemary to enhance the flavor of your food.

5. Limit Processed Foods and Sugary Drinks

Reduce your intake of processed meals, sugary snacks, refined grains, and sugary drinks, as they might worsen insulin resistance and cause inflammation.

6. Drink Plenty of Water

Drink plenty of water to stay hydrated throughout the day, and avoid alcohol and sugar-filled drinks, as they can worsen blood sugar regulation and cause inflammation.

Conclusion

Including foods that lower inflammation in your diet is a terrific strategy to improve your overall health and manage your diabetes. By reducing inflammation, these meals can improve insulin sensitivity, help stabilize blood sugar levels, and reduce the risk of complications from diabetes. A diet rich in fruits, vegetables, whole grains, lean meats, and healthy fats can help reduce inflammation by offering a range of nutrients and antioxidants. Herbs and spices such as turmeric, cinnamon, ginger, and garlic offer food flavor and reduce inflammation. By including anti-inflammatory ingredients in smoothies and juices, you can up your consumption of antioxidants and nutrients in a straightforward and revitalizing manner. Individuals who have diabetes can take control of their health and wellness by making sure to incorporate anti-inflammatory foods in their meal plans.

CHAPTER 6
MAKING NUTRIENT-PACKED MEAL PLANS

Nutrient meal planning is essential for people with diabetes to maintain blood sugar management, improve overall health, and prevent complications. Prioritizing the proper ratios of proteins, lipids, and carbohydrates is essential. A well-thought-out meal plan should also contain a variety of nutrient-dense meals and consider the person's preferences and lifestyle. This comprehensive guide includes sample menu items for breakfast, lunch, and dinner, weekly meal planning strategies, the basics of making a diabetic-friendly meal plan, tips on intelligent snacking for diabetics, the importance of staying hydrated, how to prepare meals for busy schedules, and how to adjust meal plans based on progress.

THE FUNDAMENTALS OF A DIABETES-FRIENDLY DIET

Meals rich in nutrients that promote overall health, help control blood sugar, and provide essential nutrients should take precedence in a diabetic-friendly menu.

The following considerations should be taken while designing a meal plan for people with diabetes:

1. Maintain a balance between fats, proteins, and carbs

Aim for a balance of carbohydrates, proteins, and fats at each meal to help manage blood sugar levels and provide sustained energy.

- Carbs: To lessen spikes in blood sugar levels, choose complex carbohydrates with a low glycemic index. Focus on whole grains, legumes, fruits, and vegetables.
- Proteins: Include lean protein sources such as chicken, fish, tofu, beans, and low-fat dairy to help maintain muscle mass and promote satiety.
- Fats: Select heart-healthy fats, such as those in nuts, seeds, avocados, and olive oil, to support heart health and provide essential fatty acids.

2. Place an Emphasis on Whole, Minimally Processed Foods

Prioritize complete, minimally processed foods high in nutrients and fiber, such as fruits, vegetables, whole grains, lean meats, and healthy fats.

3. Keep an eye on portion sizes.

Take note of serving sizes to help with calorie control and avoid overindulging. Use measuring cups, spoons, or visual cues to gauge portion sizes, especially for carb foods.

4. Distribute Snacks and Meals All Day

Eat regular daily meals and snacks to maintain steady blood sugar levels and prevent abrupt fluctuations.

5. Keep an eye on your blood sugar levels.

Check blood sugar levels frequently, especially after meals, to learn how different foods affect your blood sugar levels and adjust your meal plans accordingly.

STRATEGIES FOR WEEKLY MEAL PLANNING

Making a weekly food plan is a helpful approach to guarantee that you always have healthy meals and snacks available. **The following strategies might aid weekly meal planning:**

1. Schedule Planning

Momentum: Every week, schedule a specific time on a Sunday afternoon or evening to organize your meals. During this time, plan your meals for the upcoming week, make a grocery list, and review recipes.

2. Take dietary needs and personal preferences into account

When planning meals, consider your nutritional requirements, cultural influences, and personal preferences. Choose meals and recipes that satisfy your palate, dietary needs, and goals.

3. Make Well-Balanced Meal Plans

Every meal should include a sufficient amount of fruits and vegetables, along with a balance of proteins, fats, and carbohydrates. Try to make your meals as varied as possible by including a variety of textures, flavors, and colors.

4. Prepare and Cook Ingredients in Bulk

Consider bulk cooking and prepping meals to save time throughout the week. Make large quantities of meats, vegetables, and grains so you may enjoy them multiple times a week.

5. Make Use of Leftovers judiciously

Plan to use leftovers for other dinners to reduce food waste and save time. Make extra servings of food so you may store it in the fridge or utilize it in other dishes.

SAMPLE BREAKFAST, LUNCH, AND DINNER IDEAS

The following are some example meal plans for breakfast, lunch, and dinner that follow the guidelines for diabetic-friendly eating:

Breakfast:

- Vegetable Omelet: Spoon sauteed spinach, tomatoes, onions, and bell peppers into an omelet; cover with sliced avocado.
- Greek Yogurt Parfait: To add sweetness, arrange almonds, mixed berries, and honey or maple syrup on top of the Greek yogurt.
- Whole Grain bread with Nut Butter: Spread peanut butter or almond butter on the bread and then cover it with strawberries or banana slices.

Lunch:

- Quinoa salad: Mix cooked quinoa with cucumber, cherry tomatoes, chickpeas, mixed greens, and feta cheese. Toss with a lemon-juice vinaigrette.
- Turkey and Avocado Wrap: Place sliced turkey breast, avocado, lettuce, tomato, and mustard inside a whole wheat tortilla.
- Vegetables and Salmon Stir-fry: Toss salmon with bell peppers, broccoli, and snap peas, then toss it with brown rice or cauliflower rice.

Dinner:

- Roasted Vegetables with Grilled Chicken: Roast carrots, zucchini, Brussels sprouts, and grilled chicken breasts.

- Vegetable Curry: Cook a mixture of vegetables in a curry sauce made with coconut milk, ginger, and garlic. Serve the dish over brown rice.
- Stuffed Bell Peppers: Stuff cooked quinoa, black beans, corn, tomatoes, and spices into bell peppers; bake until soft.

SMART SNACKING TIPS FOR DIABETICS

An essential component of a diabetic-friendly meal plan is smart snacking, which gives you energy between meals and helps control blood sugar levels. For people with diabetes, consider these wise snacking suggestions:

1. Choose Nutrient-Dense Snacks

Choose nutrient-dense snacks like the following that offer a good ratio of fats, proteins, and carbs:
- Nut butter and fresh fruit
- Berries and Greek yogurt
- Hummus and raw veggies
- Seeds and nuts
- pineapple with cottage cheese

2. Watch Portion Sizes

Pay attention to portion sizes to prevent overindulging and consuming too many calories when snacking. Put snacks into bite-sized bags or portion-controlled containers to make snacking more convenient.

3. Plan Ahead

Make a plan and prepare food in advance to carry with you to work or when traveling. Keeping wholesome snacks close at hand can help reduce the likelihood of impulsive consumption of less healthy foods.

4. Listen to Your Body

Snack when you're hungry, not out of boredom or habit, and pay attention to your body's signals of hunger and fullness. Mindful eating can help reduce overindulgence and improve blood sugar regulation.

5. Stay Hydrated

Drink plenty of water to stay hydrated throughout the day to prevent dehydration, which can occasionally be mistaken for hunger. Stay away from sugar-filled beverages and choose water or other calorie-free liquids instead.

HYDRATION: GUIDELINES AND IMPORTANCE

Sufficient hydration is essential for overall health and well-being, particularly for people with diabetes. Maintaining adequate hydration reduces blood sugar, supports renal function, and prevents diabetes-related problems. Here are some pointers to keep you well-hydrated:

1. Consume A Lot of Water

Water is the best option for remaining hydrated; you should drink it most of the day. Attempt to drink eight glasses (64 ounces) of water or more if you're exercising or the weather is hot.

2. Keep an eye on the fluid intake.

Watch how much fluid you consume and look for signs of dehydration, such as fatigue, dark urine, dry lips, and lightheadedness. If you're exhibiting symptoms of dehydration, drink water or other liquids to replenish your fluid intake.

3. Limit Your Fluid Consumption of Sugary Drinks

Restrict the sugary beverages you drink, including sodas, fruit juices, sports drinks, and sweetened teas and coffees. If consumed in excess, these beverages can cause dehydration, increase blood sugar levels, and cause weight gain.

4. Select Drinks Without Calories

Select calorie-free beverages such as herbal tea, sparkling water, and infused water to stay hydrated without adding extra sugar or calories. These beverages could be a delightful and revitalizing option to sugar-filled ones.

5. Check the Levels of Electrolytes

For people with diabetes prone to electrolyte imbalances, it is imperative to monitor electrolyte levels and ensure enough electrolyte-rich food and beverages. To maintain electrolyte balance, consume potassium-rich foods, such as bananas, oranges, yogurt, and coconut water.

Tips for Preparing Meals for Busy Schedules

Meal prep is a helpful strategy for people with busy schedules to ensure that healthy meals are available every day of the week. Here are some meal preparation tips for people with diabetes:

1. Make a meal plan in advance.

Make time to plan your breakfast, lunch, dinner, and any extra snacks or desserts each week. Use meal plans and recipes appropriate for people with diabetes to meet your dietary goals and demands.

2. Combine ingredients in a batch and cook.

Make large quantities of meats, vegetables, and grains so you may enjoy them multiple times a week. Cooked ingredients should be stored in portion-sized containers so meals can be quickly prepared and easily accessed.

3. Utilize Kitchen Tools That Save Time

Consider investing in time-saving kitchen tools like an air fryer, Instant Pot, or slow cooker to save time when preparing and cooking meals. These appliances let you prepare meals faster and more efficiently.

4. Prepare the ingredients ahead of time.

Preparing, chopping, and washing ingredients ahead of time can save time throughout the workweek. Prepared foods can also be stored in the refrigerator in airtight, resealable bags or containers to facilitate cooking.

6. Prepare Lunches and Snacks to Go

Pack meals and snacks in bento boxes or other transportable containers on the go or at work. Preportioned and readily available meals and snacks can facilitate reducing poor food choices and impulsive eating.

Adapting Meal Plans in Light of Development

As you continue to manage your diabetes, you must regularly review and adjust your meal plan to ensure that it satisfies your nutritional needs and overall health goals. You can adjust your diet plan in light of your development by using the following advice:

1. Track Your Blood Sugar Levels

Check your blood sugar often to discover how different meals impact it, especially after eating. Look for patterns and trends over time to identify any foods or beverages that may cause fluctuations or elevations in blood sugar levels.

2. See a Registered Dietitian for advice.

Consult a qualified dietitian or certified diabetes educator for personalized guidance and support. A dietician can help you evaluate your current meal plan, make adjustments based on your preferences and development, and provide valuable advice on managing your diabetes through food.

3. Try Out Various Cuisines and Recipes

Try experimenting with different cuisines, ingredients, and cooking methods to add interest and enjoyment to your meals. Try varying your intake of fruits, vegetables, whole grains, and protein sources to improve nutritional diversity and expand your palate.

4. Modify Portion Sizes and Schedules

Adjust meal timing and serving amounts to manage blood sugar levels and promote satisfaction. Consider spacing out your meals and snacks throughout the day or adjusting the quantity of your meals based on your level of activity and hunger cues.

5. Remain adaptable and receptive.

Keep your mind open and your flexibility when changing your diet plan. Try new cuisines and cooking techniques with an open mind, and don't give up if you encounter difficulties or setbacks. Recognize your successes and focus on the process rather than the outcome as you work toward better health and wellness. Making nutrient-dense meal plans is essential to controlling diabetes because it helps patients maintain better general health, control their blood sugar levels, and prevent complications. Individuals who have diabetes can take charge of their health and well-being by following a diabetic-friendly meal plan, putting weekly meal planning techniques into practice, and savoring wholesome breakfast, lunch, and supper choices. Additionally, they can enhance their health and well-being by learning meal prep practices, eating sensibly, drinking enough water, and adjusting their meal plans in response to their progress.

Nutrition can be a pleasurable and effective way to manage diabetes, allowing those with the condition to live their best lives as long as they follow thoughtful meal plans, reliable assistance, and regular eating habits.

CHAPTER 7
PARTICULAR DIET FOR DIABETES

Food planning is essential for managing diabetes; there is no one-size-fits-all approach. Diabetes-specific diets offer several strategies for regulating blood sugar levels, promoting weight loss, and improving overall health. In this comprehensive guide, we'll look at the fundamentals, benefits, and potential downsides of plant-based diets, intermittent fasting, Paleo, and ketogenic diets. We'll also cover combining different nutritional strategies, choosing the best diet for you, and getting past health-related roadblocks.

A SYNOPSIS OF THE KETO DIET

The high-fat, low-carb diet, or ketogenic diet, induces a state of ketosis, a metabolic disorder, by promoting an eating regimen high in fat and low in carbohydrates. Typically, the diet consists of 70–80% fat, 5–10% carbohydrates, and 20–25% protein.
It functions as follows:

Method:

- Ketosis: When the body enters a state of ketosis after drastically reducing its intake of carbohydrates, it creates ketone bodies from fat storage and uses them as fuel instead of glucose.
- Insulin Sensitivity: A ketogenic diet may improve blood sugar management by reducing insulin resistance and raising insulin sensitivity.
- Weight Loss: Ketosis can help regulate obesity, a prominent risk factor for type 2 diabetes, by decreasing hunger and promoting weight loss.

Advantages:

1. Better Glycemic Control and Less Dependency on Diabetes Medications: Some research suggests that a ketogenic diet may lead to better blood sugar regulation.
2. Weight Loss: Those with diabetes who are overweight or obese may lose a significant amount of Weight by following the ketogenic diet.
3. Enhanced Energy: Many ketogenic diet adherents attest to having increased vitality and mental clarity, which may improve overall well-being.
4. Reduced Inflammation: Ketosis may have anti-inflammatory qualities that lessen the likelihood of diabetic complications.

Problems:

1. Initial adverse Effects: Often referred to as the "keto flu," this phase of going into ketosis can cause several adverse effects, including headaches, nausea, dizziness, and lethargy.
2. Nutrient Deficiencies: Because the ketogenic diet limits the number of items high in essential nutrients and high in carbohydrates, it may result in deficiencies if not strictly followed.
3. Long-Term Sustainability: Some people may find it challenging to maintain a ketosis over an extended period due to the diet's limitations and limited food selections.
4. Potential Health Risks: Long-term effects of high-fat diets on heart health are a concern, even though research in this area is still underway.

THE BENEFITS OF THE PALEO DIET

The Paleo diet, also known as the caveman or Paleolithic diet, is based on eating foods that our predecessors would have had access to during the Paleolithic era. Lean meats, fish, fruits, vegetables, nuts, and seeds are among the complete, unprocessed foods favored above grains, legumes, dairy, processed meals, and refined sugars.

It's tempting to some people with diabetes for the following reasons:

Method:

- Blood Sugar Regulation: The Paleo diet minimizes insulin resistance and stabilizes blood sugar levels by avoiding refined sugars and carbohydrates.
- Nutrient Density: The Paleo diet emphasizes whole, nutrient-dense foods, which provide essential vitamins, minerals, and antioxidants that support overall health and well-being.
- Reduction of Inflammation: Individuals with diabetes who are more prone to long-term inflammation may discover that the Paleo diet reduces inflammation.

Advantages:

1. Better Blood Sugar Control: Studies suggest that a Paleo diet may reduce HbA1c levels and better glycemic control in those with type 2 diabetes.
2. Weight Loss: People who follow the Paleo diet might lose Weight, which is beneficial for managing their diabetes because it emphasizes genuine foods and rejects processed meals.
3. Enhanced Satiety: The Paleo diet's high protein and fiber content can promote feelings of fullness and satiety, reducing the likelihood of overindulging.
4. Better Gut Health: Consuming fiber-rich fruits and vegetables can help keep your gut microbiota in good

shape and improve your digestion. The Paleo diet promotes this.

Problems:

1. Limited Food Options: The Paleo diet avoids many food groups, including dairy, legumes, and grains, which can make it challenging to get enough nutrients, especially for vegans and vegetarians.
2. Cost: The Paleo diet may be more expensive since it emphasizes premium, organic meats, seafood, and produce.
3. Social Isolation: Following a rigorous diet like the Paleo may lead to social isolation or make it difficult to go out to eat because many social gatherings revolve around foods that are not Paleo-friendly.
4. Lack of Long-Term research: Even though the preliminary results of short-term studies are favorable, more research is needed to ascertain the long-term effects of the Paleo diet on managing diabetes and overall health.

ADVANTAGES OF A DIET HIGH IN PLANTS

A plant-based diet emphasizes foods like fruits, vegetables, whole grains, legumes, nuts, and seeds sourced from plants while excluding animal products. Plant-based diets such as vegetarian, vegan, and Mediterranean emphasize the consumption of whole, minimally processed plant foods.

This is the rationale behind the standard advice to adopt a plant-based diet for diabetics:

Method:

- Enhanced Insulin Sensitivity: Plant-based diets high in protein, antioxidants, and phytochemicals can reduce the risk of type 2 diabetes and to improve insulin sensitivity.
- Weight management: Plant-based diets frequently contain fewer calories and saturated fat, which is advantageous for controlling Weight and reducing the risk of problems associated with obesity.
- Reduced Inflammation: Plant-based diets' anti-inflammatory properties can help reduce inflammation, which is a factor in insulin resistance and diabetes-related issues.

Advantages:

1. Better Glycemic Control: Research has shown that plant-based diets are associated with reduced insulin resistance and better glycemic control in individuals with diabetes.
2. Heart Health: Diabetes is associated with a lower risk of cardiovascular disease, and people with diabetes often co-occur with cardiovascular illness.
3. Weight loss: Plant-based diets can lead to significant weight loss, particularly if they emphasize whole, minimally processed foods and limit added sugars and refined carbs.
4. Lower Risk of sequelae: Plant-based diets have been associated with a lower risk of diabetic sequelae, such as neuropathy, nephropathy, and retinopathy.

Problems:

1. Nutrient Deficiencies: Plant-only diets may be deficient in critical nutrients, such as vitamin B12, calcium, iron, and omega-3 fatty acids, primarily found in animal products.
2. Protein Adequacy: Adequate protein consumption on a plant-based diet requires careful planning, especially for

individuals with higher protein requirements or those who engage in physical activity.

3. Social Stigma: If you follow a plant-based diet, you can face criticism or social stigma from others, particularly in cultures where eating meat is a firmly ingrained custom.
4. Cooking Convenience and Proficiency: Changing to a plant-based diet may require more time and effort to prepare meals. Furthermore, a wide variety of fresh fruit and plant-based products could be more accessible.

COMPREHENDING PERIODIC FASTING

Intermittent fasting (IF) is a pattern of eating in which periods of fasting and eating alternate. The two most common types of intermittent fasting are the 16/8 technique, which entails fasting for 16 hours and eating within an 8-hour window, and the 5:2 method, which entails eating regularly five days a week and restricting calories on the other two. For people with diabetes, intermittent fasting may provide the following benefits:

Method:

- Insulin Sensitivity: Intermittent fasting can potentially reduce insulin resistance and boost insulin sensitivity by promoting cellular repair processes and enhancing glucose absorption.
- Weight Loss: For people with diabetes, particularly those who are obese or overweight, intermittent fasting has the benefit of calorie restriction and weight loss.
- Autophagy: Autophagy is a process by which cells eliminate damaged or faulty components. It is brought on by fasting and can enhance metabolic health and reduce inflammation.

Advantages:

1. Better Blood Sugar Control: Studies show that intermittent fasting may improve glycemic control, decrease fasting blood sugar, and increase insulin sensitivity in individuals with type 2 diabetes.
2. Weight Loss: Intermittent fasting can lead to noticeable weight loss when combined with a healthy diet and regular exercise.
3. Flexibility and Simplicity: Some people may find intermittent fasting easier to adhere to because it doesn't require any specific foods or meal planning.
4. Metabolic Health: A few advantages of intermittent fasting for metabolic health include lowering blood pressure, improving lipid profiles, and reducing inflammation.

Problems:

1. Hypoglycemia Risk: Individuals taking certain diabetes medications, such as sulfonylureas or insulin, run the risk of developing hypoglycemia when fasting. They should so keep a careful eye on their blood sugar levels.
2. Sustainability and Adherence: Long-term intermittent fasting may be challenging, especially for people with unpredictable schedules or strong appetites.
3. Nutrient Intake: People may only consume enough nutrients during fasting periods if they eat a balanced meal during eating windows.
4. Social Implications: When fasting interferes with mealtimes and social gatherings, it could be challenging to take part in family dinners or meetings.

SELECTING THE IDEAL DIET FOR YOURSELF

When choosing the ideal diet for treating diabetes, personal preferences, lifestyle conditions, health goals, and medical factors must all be taken into account.

Consider the following aspects while selecting a diet:

1. Individual Preferences:

Consider your food choices, cultural influences, and eating habits while choosing a diet. Pick a diet that complements your tastes and way of life.

2. Objectives for Health:

Establish your health goals, which may include reducing inflammation, avoiding diabetes complications, decreasing body weight, or improving blood sugar control. Choose a diet that supports you in reaching your particular health goals.

3. Health-Related Considerations:

Be aware of any dietary restrictions or underlying medical conditions you may be experiencing, such as food allergies, gastrointestinal issues, or kidney disease. Consult a qualified dietitian or other healthcare provider for personalized guidance.

4. Durability:

Choose a diet that you will be able to maintain over the term. Avoid very strict or stringent diets as they might be challenging to stick to and lead to vitamin shortages.

5. Adaptability

Look for flexible and varied diet programs that will allow you to enjoy a wide range of meals and meet different needs, such as when traveling or attending social gatherings.

COMBINING DIETS TO GET THE BEST OUTCOMES

Sometimes combining elements of different diets can work better together to improve the control of diabetes.

Here are some examples of mixing different dietary philosophies:

1. Ketogenic Mediterranean Diet:

Combine the benefits of the Mediterranean diet—which emphasizes whole grains, fruits, vegetables, and olive oil—with the ketogenic diet's focus on high-quality fats and minimal carbohydrate intake. The combo approach may be beneficial for blood sugar control and heart health.

2. Plant-Based Paleo Diet:

Combine the Paleo diet's focus on lean meats, seafood, fruits, and vegetables with the plant-based diet's emphasis on entire, minimally processed plant foods. This combined approach provides a balanced macronutrient composition, maximizes nutrient density, and reduces inflammation.

3. Any Diet Combined with Periodic Fasting:

Any diet that incorporates intermittent fasting has the potential to maximize metabolic health, promote weight loss, and improve insulin sensitivity. Experiment with different eating times and fasting regimens to determine what works best for you.

POSSIBLE OBSTACLES AND STRATEGIES FOR GETTING PAST THEM

Diabetes-specific diets may offer some benefits, but there may also be disadvantages that patients should be aware of.

The following are some common roadblocks and strategies to get beyond them:

1. inadequacies in nutrients:

To address potential nutrient shortages, make sure your diet consists of a variety of fruits, vegetables, whole grains, lean meats, and healthy fats. Consider supplementing while working with a healthcare provider if necessary.

2. Social Detachment:

Make sure you let friends and family know what you can't eat, schedule social gatherings and eating out in advance, and select restaurants with menus that suit your needs. Focus on the company and the conversation rather than just the food.

3. Durability:

Try new recipes and meal ideas, be flexible with your diet, and find enjoyment in your food choices in order to maintain long-term sustainability. Make little, gradual changes and recognize your advancements as you go.

4. Health-Related Considerations:

For individualized help with any medical conditions or concerns, see a qualified dietician or other healthcare specialist. Be up forward and honest about your medical history, prescription medications, and dietary choices in order to receive advice that are tailored to you.

5. Emotional Consumption:

Manage your emotional eating by practicing mindful eating, identifying the circumstances that trigger overeating, and using alternative coping mechanisms like exercise, meditation, or journaling. Seek support from friends, family, or a mental health professional if needed.

Diabetes-specific specialized diets offer several approaches to regulating blood sugar, promoting weight loss, and improving overall health. Each nutritional approach has unique methods, benefits, and challenges of its own. These consist of the ketogenic diet, intermittent fasting, and plant-based diets. When choosing the optimal diet for treating diabetes, it's essential to consider sustainability, health goals, medical issues, and individual preferences.

Combining elements of different diets can improve results and work in concert to treat diabetes. The Paleo Plant-Based Diet, the Mediterranean Ketogenic Diet, or mixing intermittent fasting with any other nutritional approach are examples of hybrid dietary methods that maximize nutrient intake while providing flexibility and variety.

Diabetes diets customized for each individual may have benefits, but they may also have disadvantages. Healthcare professionals, qualified dietitians, and loved ones need to be patient, plan ahead, and provide assistance in order to address concerns such as emotional eating, social isolation, and nutritional deficiencies.

The key to effectively managing diabetes with diet is to find a balanced, long-lasting approach that fits in with lifestyle goals, personal preferences, and health goals. By exercising, eating more nutrient-dense meals, regulating portion sizes, and monitoring blood sugar levels, people can take proactive steps to improve their health and well-being.

With the advancement of knowledge about nutrition and diabetes, it is imperative to keep learning, developing, and keeping an open mind. If individuals with diabetes have the proper knowledge, tools, and mindset, they can effectively manage their diets and maintain happy, healthy lives.

CHAPTER 8
HERBAL MEDICINES AND DIETARY SUPPLEMENTS FOR DIABETES MANAGEMENT

Herbal supplements and medications work in conjunction with traditional therapies and lifestyle changes, which is crucial for the effective management of diabetes. There are plenty of solutions available for people who want to optimize their health and well-being, from essential vitamins and minerals to herbal supplements, probiotics, and prebiotics.

Safe supplementation techniques, natural diabetes management solutions, the function of probiotics and prebiotics, vitamins and minerals that are critical for diabetics, herbal supplements that help control blood sugar, how to incorporate supplements into your diet, and the importance of consulting healthcare providers are all covered in this comprehensive guide.

VITAL MINERALS AND VITAMINS FOR PEOPLE WITH DIABETES

Many metabolic processes, including insulin sensitivity, blood sugar regulation, and energy production, depend on minerals and vitamins. For people with diabetes in particular, ensuring sufficient consumption of vital nutrients is critical to maintaining overall health and lowering the risk of complications.

The following vitamins and minerals are essential for people with diabetes:

1. Vitamin D:

- Function: Vitamin D is involved in the control of inflammation, insulin sensitivity, and insulin secretion.
- The following are the sources: sun exposure, egg yolks, fortified dairy products, fatty fish (such salmon and mackerel), and dairy products.
- Supplementation: Many diabetics, particularly those with darker skin tones or infrequent sun exposure, are vitamin D deficient. It could be required to take supplements in order to reach ideal levels.

2. Magnesium:

- Function: Magnesium plays a part in blood pressure regulation, insulin action, and glucose metabolism.
- Sources include whole grains, legumes, nuts and seeds (such as almonds and pumpkin seeds), and leafy green vegetables (like spinach and kale).
- Supplementation: For some diabetics, especially those with poor food consumption or magnesium deficiencies, taking supplements of magnesium may be beneficial.

3. Chromium:

- Function: Chromium improves cellular glucose absorption and insulin sensitivity.
- Sources: Nuts, seeds, green beans, broccoli, barley, and oats.
- Supplementation: Although further studies are required to validate its effectiveness, chromium supplements may help those with type 2 diabetes achieve better glycemic control.

4. Vitamin B12:

- Role: Red blood cell formation and nerve function are both impacted by vitamin B12.

- Sources: Fortified plant-based foods (e.g., fortified nutritional yeast, fortified plant-based milk), animal products (e.g., meat, fish, dairy).
- Supplementation: People who eat a vegan or vegetarian diet may need to take supplements to prevent vitamin B12 deficiency.

5. Omega-3 Fatty Acids:
- Role: Because of their anti-inflammatory qualities, omega-3 fatty acids may lower the risk of cardiovascular disease.
- Sources: Walnuts, flaxseeds, chia seeds, and fatty fish (such as salmon, mackerel, and sardines).
- Supplementation: People with diabetes, especially those with high triglyceride levels or cardiovascular risk, may benefit from taking omega-3 supplements, such as fish oil or algal oil capsules.

HERBAL SUPPLEMENTS THAT AID BLOOD SUGAR CONTROL

Traditional medical systems have been using herbal supplements for generations to treat a variety of illnesses, including diabetes. Although studies on the effectiveness and safety of herbal supplements for managing diabetes are still in progress, certain plants have demonstrated the potential to enhance blood sugar regulation and promote general well-being. **The following herbal supplements may help with blood sugar regulation:**

1. Cinnamon:

- Mechanism: Cinnamon may increase cellular absorption of glucose and insulin sensitivity.
- Dosage: 1 to 6 grams of cinnamon per day have been used in studies.
- Forms: Cinnamon can be taken as a supplement in the form of capsules or extract, or it can be used as a spice in food and drinks.

2. Fenugreek:

- Mechanism: Soluble fiber and chemicals included in fenugreek seeds have the potential to reduce blood sugar levels and enhance insulin sensitivity.
- Doses of fenugreek seeds ranging from 2.5 to 25 grams per day have been utilized in studies.
- Forms: Fenugreek can be taken as a supplement, as whole seeds, or as powdered seeds.

3. Gymnema Sylvestre:

- Mechanism: Gymnema Sylvestre may enhance pancreatic insulin synthesis while decreasing intestinal absorption of sugar.
- Dosage: Gymnema Sylvestre extract has been utilized in studies at levels of 200–800 mg per day.
- Forms: A standardized extract is the most common supplement form of Gymnema Sylvestre.

4. Bitter Melon:

- Mechanism: Compounds in bitter melon may lower blood sugar and enhance insulin sensitivity.
- Dosage: 50–100 milliliters of bitter melon juice or 2–3 grams of bitter melon powder per day have been utilized in studies.

- Forms: Bitter melon can be taken as a supplement, vegetable, or juice.

5. Ginseng:
- Mechanism: Ginseng has the potential to enhance glucose metabolism and insulin sensitivity.
- Dosage: 200–3,000 mg of ginseng extract per day have been used in studies.
- Forms: There are several ways to consume ginseng, including as tablets, capsules, extracts, and teas.

6. Berberine:
- Mechanism: By enhancing insulin sensitivity and decreasing insulin resistance, berberine may help reduce blood sugar levels.
- Dosage: 500–1,500 mg of berberine per day have been used in studies.
- Forms: Standardized extracts of berberine are commonly sold as supplements.

7. Aloe Vera:
- Mechanism: By increasing insulin sensitivity and lowering fasting blood sugar levels, aloe vera may help with blood sugar regulation.
- Dosage: Aloe vera extract doses in studies have ranged from 300 to 1,000 mg daily.
- Forms: Aloe vera comes in a number of forms, such as juice, gel, and supplements.

THE ROLE OF PROBIOTICS AND PREBIOTICS

Prebiotics are indigestible fibers that provide probiotics—beneficial microorganisms that promote gut health—with nourishment. Together, probiotics and prebiotics promote a healthy gut flora, which may influence metabolic pathways linked to diabetes and have implications for overall health. **Here are several ways that probiotics and prebiotics can aid in the treatment of diabetes:**

Probiotics:

- Mechanism: Probiotics may improve insulin sensitivity, reduce inflammation, and change the flora in the stomach.
- Sources: Probiotics can be found in fermented foods, including kombucha, yogurt, kefir, sauerkraut, and kimchi.
- Supplementation: Probiotic supplements come in a variety of strains and formulations, some of which may be advantageous to people with diabetes.

Prebiotics:

- Mechanism: Prebiotics support the growth of beneficial bacteria in the stomach by feeding probiotics.
- Sources: Prebiotics can be found in foods like bananas, chicory root, garlic, onions, leeks, and asparagus.
- Supplementation: Prebiotic supplements can be taken in a variety of forms, including powders, capsules, and functional meals.

Safe Practices for Supplementation

Supplements may be beneficial for diabetics, but it's crucial to put safety first and proceed with caution.

Take into account the following secure supplementation methods:

1. Speak with Healthcare Professionals:

- Before starting any new supplement regimen, make sure it is appropriate for your particular health needs and medical history by consulting a competent nutritionist or your healthcare practitioner.

2. Select Premium Supplements:

- Select dietary supplements from reputable producers who subject their goods to impartial testing to guarantee their strength, quality, and purity.

3. Begin Gradually and Track the Results:

- Introduce nutrition gradually and monitor your body's response. Watch out for any adverse effects or interactions with medications.

4. Pay Attention to Doses:

- Follow the dose guidelines provided by healthcare providers or the supplement's maker. Unless a healthcare practitioner instructs you otherwise, you should not go over recommendations.

5. Think about how nutrients interact:

- Identify the potential for interactions between medications and supplements. Discussing possible interactions with your healthcare provider is crucial because several supplements have the potential to alter how well medications function or are absorbed.

6. Track Nutrient Amounts:

- Make sure supplements are meeting your needs and not causing imbalances or deficiencies by regularly monitoring your blood levels through blood tests.

NATURAL DIABETES MANAGEMENT TECHNIQUES

Together with supplements and herbal medications, a number of natural therapies may help improve overall health and support the control of diabetes. These include dietary modifications, techniques for reducing stress, lifestyle modifications, and complementary therapies.

Take into consideration these natural remedies:

1. Exercise:

- Frequent exercise can improve insulin sensitivity, blood sugar control, and weight management. Combine cardiovascular, flexibility, and strength training routines for optimal results.

2. Reducing Stress:

- Prolonged stress may worsen insulin resistance and blood sugar problems. Take part in stress-relieving exercises such as yoga, tai chi, mindfulness meditation, deep breathing, and outdoor activities.

3. Suitable Sleep Position:

- Prioritize obtaining adequate sleep in order to enhance overall wellness and metabolism. Make the most of your sleeping environment, establish a peaceful bedtime routine, and stick to a regular sleep schedule in order to achieve your goal of seven to nine hours of uninterrupted sleep each night.

4. Consciously Consuming Food:

- Practice mindful eating by paying attention to your body's cues about hunger and fullness, chewing your food thoroughly and slowly, and savoring its flavors and textures. Mindful eating has been shown to improve nutrient absorption, enhance meal satisfaction, and improve digestion.

5. Herbal Teas:

- Certain herbal teas, such as green tea, hibiscus, and chamomile, may help lower blood sugar, oxidative stress, and inflammation. Herbal teas are hydrating and can provide a host of other health benefits if you incorporate them into your daily regimen.

How to Include Supplements in Your Meal Plan

Including supplements in your diet requires careful planning and consideration of individual requirements and preferences.

You can incorporate vitamins into your everyday regimen by using the following advice:

1. Create a Schedule:

- Include supplements in your daily routine by taking them at the same time each day, such as with breakfast or supper. You can make it easier to remember to bring your supplements on time by using pill organizers or setting reminders.

2. Select User-Friendly Forms:

- Select supplements for your diet in forms that are easy to mix and convenient, including powders, tablets, or capsules. Consider factors including flavor, texture, and ease of ingestion while choosing supplements.

3. Match with Meals:

- Take supplements with meals or snacks to enhance absorption and reduce the risk of stomach distress. Certain supplements may be absorbed more readily when consumed with foods heavy in fat or protein.

4. Keep an eye on the effects:

- Monitor how your body responds to supplements and adjust your regimen as needed. If you have any adverse reactions or interactions, consult your physician immediately.

5. Maintain Hydration:

- Drink lots of water throughout the day to stay hydrated and absorb water-soluble vitamins and minerals. Sustaining proper hydration is essential for overall health and wellness.

Advising Medical Providers

Before making any significant dietary or supplement changes, you should always see a healthcare provider so they can provide you with personalized guidance and assistance.

It's critical to speak with healthcare providers for the following reasons:

1. Personalized Suggestions:

- Healthcare specialists can assess your medical history, current prescriptions, and unique health needs to make personalized recommendations for supplements.

2. Observation and Assessment:
- Medical practitioners can monitor your growth, perform vitamin tests on your blood, and ascertain the long-term effects of supplements on your health.

3. Safety Observations:
- Medical practitioners are qualified to help you navigate the risks, interactions, and contraindications associated with supplements, ensuring your regimen is safe and appropriate for your current health status.

4. Comprehensive Method:
- Healthcare experts manage diabetes using a comprehensive strategy that considers medicine, lifestyle, diet, and supplementation to construct comprehensive treatment plans tailored to your individual goals and needs.

5. Responsibility and Assistance:
- Healthcare experts are trustworthy allies and resources when attempting to get healthier. They can motivate, inspire, and guide you to stick to your diet and supplement regimens.

Herbal medications and supplements improve insulin sensitivity, blood sugar regulation, and overall health, greatly aiding diabetes management. Essential vitamins and minerals, such as vitamin D, magnesium, chromium, and omega-3 fatty acids, are required to maintain a healthy metabolism and lower the risk of diabetes-related issues. The effectiveness and safety of herbal supplements containing cinnamon, fenugreek, and bitter melon, which have shown promise in enhancing insulin sensitivity and blood sugar levels, need further investigation.

Probiotics and prebiotics are critical for preserving gut health, which is becoming recognized as essential for diabetes management. Probiotics can help manage the gut microbiome, reduce inflammation, and improve insulin sensitivity, while prebiotics function as food for healthy gut bacteria, promoting their growth and activity.

When incorporating supplements into your diet, you must prioritize safety and consult a healthcare provider to ensure the supplements are appropriate for your unique goals and needs. Reduce risks and maximize benefits by taking good care of yourself initially, using premium supplements, and monitoring your progress over time. In addition to supplements, herbal teas, mindful eating, stress reduction techniques, and physical activity are natural therapies that can help with dietary and lifestyle modifications for diabetes control.

These comprehensive approaches improve overall metabolic function and promote long-term fitness by addressing every aspect of health and wellness. Ultimately, managing diabetes requires a comprehensive approach that includes dietary changes, lifestyle modifications, medication administration, and, on occasion, vitamin, mineral, and herbal supplements.

By working closely with healthcare professionals, people with diabetes can design personalized treatment plans that address their unique needs, optimize metabolic health, and improve quality of life. In conclusion, using vitamins and herbal remedies can be very beneficial for those seeking to improve their general health and well-being and adequately control their diabetes.

By integrating probiotics, prebiotics, essential vitamins, minerals, and herbal supplements into their diet, people with diabetes can improve their insulin sensitivity, reduce their risk of complications from the disease, and support blood sugar control.

It is essential to approach supplementation cautiously, prioritize safety, and consult with healthcare specialists to ensure that supplements are appropriate and beneficial for specific health requirements and goals. With careful planning, thorough supervision, and support from medical specialists, people with diabetes can use herbal medicines and supplements to optimize their health and survive despite the challenges of the illness.

CHAPTER 9
ADVANCES IN LIFESTYLE TO HELP MANAGEMENT OF DIABETES

Diabetes treatment necessitates a multifaceted approach that extends beyond dietary modifications and prescription medication. Lifestyle adjustments are necessary for people with diabetes to control their blood sugar, reduce their risk of complications, and improve their overall health. This comprehensive book will address a wide range of subjects, such as the importance of regular exercise, strategies for reducing stress, improving sleep quality, mindfulness and meditation practices, building a support system, implementing long-term lifestyle changes, and tracking and monitoring outcomes.

THE SIGNIFICANCE OF FREQUENT EXERCISE

Physical activity is the cornerstone of diabetic management and offers numerous physical and mental health benefits. Regular exercise can reduce cardiovascular risk factors, assist weight control, lower blood sugar, improve insulin sensitivity, and enhance overall quality of life.

Physical activity is crucial for diabetics for the following reasons:

1. Increases Sensitivity to Insulin:

- After physical activity, the body becomes more responsive to insulin, facilitating the absorption and utilization of glucose from the bloodstream by cells for energy production. This may lower blood sugar levels and reduce the need for insulin or other prescription medications.

2. Reduces Levels of Blood Sugar:

- Increased muscle absorption of glucose during exercise can lead to sharp reductions in blood sugar levels during and after physical activity. Regular exercise improves long-term glycemic regulation, which reduces the risk of hyperglycemia and its associated complications.

3. Helps With Weight Management

- Exercise is essential for controlling Weight in individuals with diabetes, particularly those who are overweight or obese. It increases metabolism, burns calories, and develops lean muscle mass. Maintaining a healthy weight can improve insulin sensitivity and reduce the risk of type 2 diabetes complications.

4. Lowers the Risk of Cardiovascular Disease:

- Diabetes is a significant risk factor for cardiovascular disease. Regular exercise improves cholesterol, lowers blood pressure, strengthens the heart and blood vessels, and reduces inflammation. All of these advantages reduce the risk of heart attacks, strokes, and other cardiovascular events.

5. Improves Emotion and Health:

- Exercise causes the release of endorphins, which are neurotransmitters that elevate feelings of happiness and well-being. Frequent exercise can help people with diabetes feel better overall, reduce stress, worry, and sadness, and enhance their sleep quality.

To get the benefits of physical activity, aim for at least 150 minutes of moderate-intensity aerobic exercise every week, spread out across at least three days, with no more than two days off in between. Incorporate a variety of your preferred exercises, such as weightlifting, cycling, walking, swimming, dancing, or other sports. Consult a healthcare provider before starting a new exercise regimen, particularly if you have any underlying medical conditions.

TECHNIQUES FOR STRESS MANAGEMENT

As stress can significantly impact blood sugar levels and general health, managing stress is essential to managing diabetes. Prolonged stress can result in the release of stress hormones like cortisol and adrenaline, which can boost blood sugar and lead to weight gain, insulin resistance, and an increased risk of cardiovascular disease. People with diabetes can improve their overall health and control their blood sugar levels more effectively by learning effective stress management techniques. **Think about implementing these stress-reduction techniques:**

1. Breathing Techniques:

- Deep breathing exercises, such as diaphragmatic or belly breathing, can help initiate the body's relaxation response, which reduces stress and promotes calmness.

2. Meditation with mindfulness:

- Through mindfulness meditation, you can analyze your thoughts and feelings more clearly and acceptably by focusing your attention on the present moment without passing judgment. Regular mindfulness practice reduces stress, anxiety, and depressive symptoms, improving overall mental health and well-being.

3. Progressive Relaxation of the Muscles:

- Progressive muscle relaxation promotes relaxation and helps reduce physical stress by tensing and relaxing different body muscular groups. This technique can reduce stress levels, stiffness and tightness in the muscles, and the quality of sleep.

4. Tai Chi and Yoga:

- Yoga and Tai Chi are mind-body practices that combine physical postures, breathing exercises, and meditation techniques to improve balance, flexibility, and relaxation. These methods can help people with diabetes feel better overall, reduce stress, and elevate their mood.

5. Hobbies and Activities Engaged:

- Engaging in pleasurable hobbies and endeavors can serve as a pleasant diversion from pressures, aid in decompression, and help you form relationships with people who share your interests.

Stress management techniques can improve your general quality of life, reduce stress's harmful effects on your health, and help you more skillfully deal with the challenges of having diabetes.

ENHANCING THE QUALITY OF SLEEP FOR BETTER HEALTH

Even though adequate sleep is essential for overall health and wellness, many people with diabetes struggle with insomnia and other sleep disorders. Sleep deprivation is critical to diabetes treatment because it impairs insulin sensitivity, appetite regulation, blood sugar regulation, and cardiovascular health. **People with diabetes can gain from improved sleep in the following ways:**

1. control levels of blood sugar:

- A healthy sleep schedule improves glucose metabolism and insulin sensitivity, contributing to blood sugar regulation. Long-term sleep loss increases the likelihood of insulin resistance, elevated cortisol levels, and decreased glucose tolerance, all of which are linked to type 2 diabetes complications and hyperglycemia.

2. Aids in Weight Management

- Sleep is necessary to regulate hunger and preserve energy balance. Lack of sleep can disrupt hunger-related hormones like ghrelin and leptin, leading to an increase in appetite, desire for high-calorie foods, and weight gain. Individuals with diabetes who prioritize getting enough sleep are more adept at managing their Weight and less likely to suffer the negative effects of obesity.

3. Enhances Mental and Mood Health:

- Sleep is essential for mental health, emotional regulation, and cognitive performance. Chronic sleep deprivation has been associated with mood disorders such as sadness and anxiety, which can exacerbate stress and negatively impact diabetes management. Emphasizing restorative sleep can improve mood, cognitive function, and overall mental health in people with diabetes.

4. Boosts Immune Response:

- The immune system's function depends on sleep, strengthening the body's resistance to illnesses and infections. Long-term sleep loss lowers immunity, increasing susceptibility to infections and inflammatory diseases, exacerbating diabetes-related problems.

5. Encourages Recuperation and Healing:

- While you sleep, the body undergoes essential processes of regeneration and repair that support general healing, tissue repair, and muscle growth. Restorative sleep is essential for people with diabetes, who may be more vulnerable to repercussions like diabetic neuropathy and diabetic foot ulcers. It is also necessary for wound healing, glycogen replenishment, and recovery from physical and psychological stress.

If you want to improve the quality of your sleep, make good sleep hygiene a priority. This includes arranging your sleeping area, creating a peaceful nighttime routine, adhering to a regular sleep schedule, and avoiding stimulants like gadgets and coffee right before bed. If your sleep issues persist, consult a physician to determine the cause and research potential remedies such as medication or cognitive-behavioral therapy for insomnia.

PRACTICES OF MINDFULNESS AND MEDITATION

Mindfulness and meditation are valuable tools for lowering stress, promoting relaxation, and enhancing overall well-being in people with diabetes. While mindfulness involves paying attention to the present moment with openness, curiosity, and acceptance, meditation concentrates on a specific object, concept, or sensation to increase awareness and concentration. By helping patients manage the challenges brought on by their condition, both strategies can improve the quality of life for those with diabetes.

Patients with diabetes can gain from mindfulness and meditation activities in the following ways:

1. Reducing Stress:

- Mindfulness and meditation activities can improve stress management and mental health in those with diabetes by promoting relaxation and reducing the body's stress reaction.

2. Blood Sugar Regulation:

- Studies have shown that mindfulness-based treatments can improve blood sugar management in diabetics and reduce hemoglobin A1c levels. Mindfulness practices can lower blood glucose levels by promoting emotional equilibrium and reducing stress.

3. Controlling Weight:

- Mindful eating is one facet of mindfulness practice that encourages individuals to be conscious of their eating patterns, preferences, and hunger cues. By understanding and accepting their eating habits nonjudgmentally, patients with diabetes can manage portion sizes, avoid emotional eating, and select healthier foods.

4. Enhanced Quality of Sleep:

- Those who practice mindfulness meditation, which can help them relax and slow their racing thoughts, may find it easier to fall asleep and stay asleep. By including mindfulness practices in their evening routine, people can enhance their overall sleep hygiene and sleep quality.

5. Improved Emotional Health:

- By practicing mindfulness and meditation, people with diabetes can strengthen their sense of emotional resilience, acceptance, and self-compassion. By developing a positive mindset and reducing negative thinking, people can improve their overall quality of life and better handle the challenges of having a chronic condition.

Start incorporating mindfulness and meditation practices into your daily routine with short guided meditation sessions or mindfulness activities. You can use online resources, classes, workshops, and mindfulness software to learn more about different meditation techniques and how to incorporate them in your life.

Try to be mindful of the present moment by pausing, breathing, and being in the present moment when doing regular activities like eating, walking, or cleaning dishes.

ESTABLISHING A NETWORK OF SUPPORT

For those who have diabetes, building a solid support system is essential because it provides them with emotional, practical, and social support. At the same time, they navigate the challenges posed by their illness. A support system can include friends, family, healthcare providers, diabetes educators, support groups, online forums, and support groups.

The value of a support network in managing diabetes is justified by the following:

1. Psychological Assistance:

- Living with diabetes can be emotionally exhausting, resulting in stress, anxiety, dread, and frustration. A support system provides a safe space to express your emotions, seek validation, and receive encouragement and understanding from those who understand your circumstances.

2. Helpful Advice:

- Essential components of controlling diabetes include checking blood sugar levels, adhering to prescription schedules, adjusting to significant lifestyle changes, and navigating healthcare institutions. A support system can assist with things like meal planning, exercise routines, medication reminders, and doctor's appointments to help relieve the burden of self-management responsibilities.

3. Knowledge and Instruction:

- A support network can provide valuable information, resources, and educational materials about managing diabetes, available therapies, lifestyle modifications, and local services. By sharing information, people can stay informed about the latest developments in diabetes care, gain from one another's knowledge and experiences, and make well-informed decisions about their health.

4. Relationship with Others:

- Sometimes, having diabetes might make you feel isolated, especially if you don't have many people in your support network. Forming connections with those who also have diabetes can lessen feelings of loneliness and foster social connection and camaraderie by providing a sense of understanding, solidarity, and belonging.

5. Drive and Responsibility:

- People struggling to maintain their diabetes control goals might find motivation, accountability, and encouragement from their support system. Whether it's a cooking partner, workout partner, or peer mentor, having someone to talk to about successes, setbacks, and progress can help maintain motivation and long-term habit modification.

Identify a support system by contacting friends, family, healthcare providers, or local diabetic support groups. In addition, you can participate in social media groups and online forums devoted to diabetes management, where you can receive advice, encouragement, and support from those who have experienced the same circumstances. Building a support system takes time and effort, so be patient and considerate as you build strong relationships with people.

MAKING A CHANGE IN LIFESTYLE THAT IS SUSTAINABLE

Diabetes management requires long-term lifestyle changes and a commitment to maintaining better habits. Rather than focusing on short fixes or drastic measures, make small, sustainable changes that fit your hobbies, lifestyle, and values.

Here's how to modify your lifestyle permanently to manage your diabetes:

1. Establish sensible objectives:

- Before you start, make sure your goals are realistic, reachable, and consistent with your abilities, priorities, and preferences. Divide more ambitious objectives into more minor, manageable activities and celebrate your progress to stay inspired and involved.

2. Emphasize changing behavior:

- Prioritize practices and behavior changes that improve overall health and well-being over outcomes like blood sugar control or weight loss. Find out exactly what actions you can take to enhance the quality of your sleep, lower your stress level, get more exercise, and make dietary improvements.

3. Locate Pleasurable Activities:

- Choose activities and physical endeavors you enjoy, including hiking, gardening, dancing to your favorite music, or participating in sports. Add variety and freshness to your routine to keep things interesting and prevent burnout or boredom.

4. Exercise Self-Compassion:

- As you navigate the highs and lows of managing your diabetes, treat yourself with respect and understanding. Construct a tough, tenacious, and self-accepting mindset by seeing challenges and disappointments as opportunities for growth.

5. Seek Expert Assistance:

- Asking medical professionals, registered dietitians, diabetic educators, counselors, or other specialists for their professional advice is never a sign of weakness. They can provide you with guidance, responsibility, and individualized counsel to assist you in achieving your health goals.

6. Make Modest Adjustments:

- Aim to make little, sustainable changes to your lifestyle over time rather than trying to overhaul your routine entirely at once. Start with one or two habits at a time, such as adding a portion of vegetables to your meals or taking a brisk walk after dinner, and work your way up to more.

7. Remain Adaptive and Flexible:

- Keep an open mind and be prepared to adjust your plan and direction when needed in reaction to your body's signals, new information, or situations. Stay flexible, adaptive, and willing to test different strategies until you find the one that works best for you.

KEEPING AN EYE ON AND TRACKING YOUR DEVELOPMENT

Monitoring your progress is essential to assess how well your diabetes management strategies are working, identify areas that need improvement, and sustain your motivation to reach your goals. By frequently monitoring key indicators like blood sugar levels, physical activity, nutritional consumption, and mental well-being, you can gain valuable insights into how your lifestyle choices affect your health and make well-informed decisions regarding modifications and adaptations.

Here's how to effectively keep tabs on and assess your development:

1. Maintain a Diabetes Diary:

- Keep a diabetic journal or logbook to record important information such as blood sugar readings, medication dosages, meals and snacks, physical activity, stress, sleep patterns, and mood swings. By looking back through your diary entries over time, you can identify trends, patterns, and triggers that may impact how you manage your diabetes.

2. Utilize technological instruments:

- Utilize modern resources such as blood glucose meters, fitness trackers, continuous glucose monitors (CGMs), and smartphone apps to manage your diabetes effectively. These technologies can provide real-time data, insights, and feedback to help you make well-informed decisions about your health. Use them to record food intake, monitor your exercise, monitor blood sugar levels, set up medication dose reminders, and receive personalized guidance based on your needs and goals.

3. Make Measurable Objectives:

- Establish measurable, specific goals for managing your diabetes, such as reaching your target blood sugar range, increasing your physical activity, improving your diet, controlling your stress levels, or improving your sleep. Break down more challenging goals into more doable benchmarks, and keep a close eye on your progress to stay motivated and accountable.

4. Track Your Blood Sugar Levels:

- Use a blood glucose meter or continuous glucose monitor (CGM) to check your blood sugar levels as your healthcare provider prescribes. Throughout the day, monitor your readings and record any trends or deviations. Inform your medical staff of your findings so that any required adjustments can be made to your treatment plan.

5. Monitor Your Exercise:

- Keep a journal of your workouts, recording the type, duration, degree of difficulty, and frequency of your physical activity. Set weekly or monthly targets for physical exercise and track your progress over time. Gradually extend or intensify your workouts as your level of fitness rises.

6. Track your food intake:

- Using a food journal or a smartphone app, track your nutritional intake, including meals, snacks, portion sizes, and macronutrient makeup. Pay attention to the number and quality of your meals and the amount of carbs you eat to support adequate blood sugar regulation. Make any necessary adjustments.

7. Determine Stress Levels:

- Monitor your emotional and stress levels regularly. Look for signs of stress such as fatigue, irritability, tenseness in your muscles, or difficulty concentrating. Use relaxation techniques, stress management strategies, and self-care routines to promote emotional balance and lessen stress.

8. Assess the Quality of Your Sleep:

- Use a sleep journal or tracker to assess the duration and caliber of your sleep, the times you go to bed and wake up, and any disturbances or issues that arise during the night. Aim for seven to nine hours of restorative sleep per night. If necessary, you can improve the quality of your sleep by adjusting your sleeping environment or ritual before bed.

9. Consider Your Progress:

- Remember your victories, challenges, and accomplishments in coping with your diabetes. Acknowledge successes, learn from setbacks, identify areas for improvement, and see every experience as an opportunity for personal growth.

10. Interact with Healthcare Professionals:

- Talk to your healthcare providers about monitoring data, progress, and concerns during regular check-ups or appointments. Discuss any changes in your health status, treatment choices, or lifestyle habits with your healthcare team so that personalized goals and action plans can be developed for the best possible management of your diabetes.

Regularly tracking and recording your progress will help you get valuable insights into your diabetes management efforts, identify areas for improvement, and make well-informed decisions about changing your treatment plan or lifestyle.

Continue to be proactive, engaged, and committed to your health goals. Remember that even small changes can lead to progressive improvements in your overall health. A person's physical, mental, and emotional well-being can be significantly enhanced by making lifestyle changes, which are also essential for effective diabetes management.

By adopting regular physical activity, stress management techniques, improved sleep hygiene, mindfulness and meditation practices, creating a support system, making sustainable lifestyle changes, and monitoring their progress, people with diabetes can take control of their health and enhance their quality of life.

Remember that managing diabetes is a journey rather than a one-size-fits-all approach. A personalized treatment plan that considers your individual needs and goals can be created by experimenting with different strategies, paying close attention to your body, and working with your medical team.

Maintain your proactive, persistent, and committed approach to managing your diabetes, and remember to celebrate your small victories along the way. Despite the challenges posed by diabetes, you can succeed and enjoy a long, healthy life if you are persistent, dedicated, and have support.

CHAPTER 10
TESTIMONIALS AND SUCCESS STORIES IN THE TREATMENT OF DIABETES

Learning from the experiences of others can be pretty illuminating and inspirational, especially when it comes to managing a complex illness like diabetes. Testimonials and success stories provide valuable, real-world examples of people who have overcome challenges, made lifestyle changes, and experienced excellent outcomes in successfully managing their diabetes. This comprehensive guide will look at six exciting case studies demonstrating different approaches to managing diabetes, including nutritional interventions, lifestyle changes, and additional tactics.

CASE STUDY 1: JOHN'S PATH TO DIABETES TYPE 2 REVERSAL

John, a 55-year-old man with type 2 diabetes, is determined to reverse his condition after experiencing problems with obesity, excessive medication use, and high blood sugar. As part of his deliberate effort to take control of his health, John embraced a holistic approach that included regular physical activity, stress management techniques, and dietary adjustments.

Dietary Adjustments:

John changed to a low-carb, high-fiber diet focused on complete, nutrient-dense meals, including vegetables, fruits, lean meats, and healthy fats. He ate meals that supported stable blood sugar levels and balanced macronutrients, consuming fewer processed foods, sweetened beverages, and refined carbohydrates.

Frequent Exercise:

John included strength training, flexibility training, and brisk walking in his daily routine. He tried to get in at least thirty minutes of moderate-intensity aerobic activity most days of the week. He gradually increased the duration and intensity of his workouts as his fitness level rose.

Techniques for Stress Management:

After learning that stress has a detrimental impact on blood sugar regulation, John began implementing stress-reduction tactics such as mindfulness meditation, deep breathing exercises, and relaxation methods. He believed that hobbies, self-care, and social connections were highly valuable in reducing stress and improving mental health.

CASE STUDY2: MARIA'S PLANT-BASED DIET SUCCESS

Maria, a 40-year-old type 2 diabetic, discovered that eating a plant-based diet rich in fruits, vegetables, whole grains, legumes, and nuts greatly improved her ability to control her condition. Driven by the benefits of a plant-based diet in treating diabetes, Maria made a significant dietary change that restored her health.

Plant-Based Diet:

Maria switched to a plant-based diet high in fiber, vitamins, minerals, and phytonutrients and mainly comprised of whole, minimally processed foods. She centered her meals on plant-based protein sources such as beans, lentils, tofu, and tempeh and consumed colorful fruits and vegetables.

Blood Sugar Regulation:

Maria stabilized her blood sugar levels and reduced her reliance on diabetic medication by prioritizing plant-based diets with high fiber content and low glycemic index values. Her blood glucose varied less, her insulin sensitivity increased, and her overall metabolic health improved.

Controlling Weight:

Maria was able to achieve and sustain a healthy weight by switching to a plant-based diet because plant-based foods generally include more fiber and fewer calories than animal-based meals. She experienced no deprivation or hunger pangs as she lost Weight gradually and persistently, which enhanced her body composition and metabolic efficiency.

CASE STUDY 3: MARK'S KETOGENIC DIET-RELATED METABOLIC CHANGE

Mark, a 45-year-old man with type 2 diabetes and obesity, saw a significant improvement in his health when he began following a ketogenic diet that is very low in carbohydrates, moderate in protein, and high in fat. Although Mark was initially dubious, he experienced noticeable improvements in his health indices and was able to consistently lose Weight by adhering to a ketogenic diet.

Nutrition for Ketosis:

Mark followed a ketogenic diet that restricted his daily carbohydrate intake to less than 50 grams. He consumed more healthy fats from foods like avocados, nuts, seeds, olive oil, and fatty fish. Mark's body entered a state of ketosis, which caused rapid weight loss and improved metabolic health, switching from using glucose as fuel to burning fat for energy.

Regulation of Blood Sugar:

One of the most notable benefits of the ketogenic diet for Mark was improved blood sugar management. By cutting back on carbohydrates and normalizing his insulin levels, Mark was able to lower his risk of blood glucose spikes and crashes. As a result of the improved glycemic control, his requirement for diabetic medicine was reduced.

Loss of Weight:

Following a ketogenic diet helped Mark shed a significant amount of body fat and reduced his risk of developing obesity-related diseases such as metabolic syndrome and cardiovascular disease. Over time, Mark discovered that the high-fat, low-carb nature of the ketogenic diet made it easier to follow his eating plan.

CASE STUDY 4: EMMA'S INTERMITTENT FASTING EXPERIENCE

Emma, a 35-year-old woman with prediabetes and insulin resistance, researched the benefits of intermittent fasting as a strategy to improve her metabolic health and prevent type 2 diabetes. She found that including intermittent fasting in her practice helped her overall well-being, insulin sensitivity, and blood sugar control.

Protocol for Intermittent Fasting:

Emma experimented with various intermittent fasting methods, including eating within a specific time frame, fasting every other day, and occasionally going longer than usual. She started by adhering to a 16:8 fasting schedule, which required her to fast for 16 hours the night before and then eat all her meals within an 8-hour window. With the assistance of a healthcare professional, she steadily increased the window of time she could fast and included extended fasting durations, such as 24-hour or multi-day fasts.

An increase in insulin sensitivity:

Emma's intermittent fasting increased her cells' ability to use glucose and regulate blood sugar levels by increasing her sensitivity to insulin. Fasting periods she helped to reduce insulin resistance and levels of the hormone insulin, which in turn helped to stabilize blood sugar levels and lessen the need for diabetic medication.

Improved Fat Loss:

By implementing intermittent fasting, Emma was able to reduce her body weight and improve her metabolic flexibility. This allowed her body to switch more easily between burning fat and glucose for energy. Emma used the fat that her body had stored during fasting periods to lose Weight gradually and sustainably. Visceral obesity is one of the main risk factors for type 2 diabetes and cardiovascular disease.

Autophagy and the Repair of Cells:

Intermittent fasting triggered autophagy, a cellular cleaning system that removes damaged or defective parts and promotes cellular repair and regeneration. This natural cleansing process regenerated Emma's cells, tissues, and organs, extending her life and improving her general health.

CASE STUDY 5: USING ANTI-INFLAMMATORY FOODS TO AID LINDA'S RECOVERIES

Linda, a fifty-year-old woman, has type 2 diabetes and chronic inflammation. She consumed a diet rich in whole, plant-based foods and immune-stimulating minerals to regain her health. By reducing inflammation and encouraging her body's natural healing processes, Linda experienced significant improvements in her general health and control of her diabetes.

Anti-Inflammatory Diet:

Linda created an anti-inflammatory diet with antioxidants like fruits, vegetables, leafy greens, berries, nuts, seeds, fatty fish, olive oil, and anti-inflammatory spices like turmeric, ginger, and garlic. She ate fewer foods that induce inflammation, such as processed meat, refined sugar, trans fats, and artificial additives.

Decreased Inflammation:

Through dietary changes, Linda's body demonstrated a lowered overall level of inflammation as seen by decreases in inflammatory indicators such as C-reactive protein (CRP) and interleukin-6 (IL-6). After treating the underlying cause of inflammation, Linda's body became more resilient to oxidative stress, immunological dysfunction, and chronic illness.

Blood Sugar Regulation:

The anti-inflammatory diet helped Linda's blood sugar levels stabilize and her insulin resistance reduce, making it easier for her to manage her diabetes without using too many prescription medications. Anti-inflammatory meals promoted hormonal balance and metabolic harmony, allowing Linda's body to better regulate insulin release and blood glucose levels.

Boosted Immune Response:

By consuming foods and supplements that stimulate the immune system, Linda improved her body's ability to fight infections, infection-causing agents, and environmental toxins. Individuals with diabetes require a robust immune system due to their potential increased susceptibility to infections and related complications.

CASE STUDY 6: DAVID'S NARRATIVE OF INTEGRATING SUPPLEMENTS AND DIETS

David, a sixty-year-old man, treated his type 2 diabetes and metabolic syndrome by combining specific supplementation strategies with dietary treatments. By addressing underlying nutritional deficiencies and increasing his food intake, David significantly improved his quality of life and health.

Nutritional Interventions:

David followed a specially designed diet that combined elements of the Mediterranean diet, low-carbohydrate eating, and intermittent fasting. He favored nutrient-dense, whole foods, including fruits, vegetables, legumes, nuts, seeds, whole grains, lean proteins, and healthy fats, and reduced his intake of processed foods, sugar-filled beverages, and refined carbohydrates.

Specific Supplementation:

In addition to dietary adjustments, David supplemented with vital vitamins, minerals, and herbal remedies that enhance insulin sensitivity, blood sugar management, and general metabolic health. These included cinnamon, alpha-lipoic acid, magnesium, chromium, berberine, vitamin D, and other nutrients good for diabetes.

All-encompassing Method:

David treated his diabetes holistically, treating the underlying imbalances and deficiencies that contributed to it rather than just taking medication to treat its symptoms. He worked closely with physicians to monitor his progress, adjust his course of therapy, and improve his long-term well-being.

CONCLUSION

These case studies highlight the range of approaches to diabetes management and the potential advantages of dietary changes, supplementation regimens, and lifestyle improvements. Since each person's journey is unique, what works for one person might not work for another.

Nevertheless, these testimonials and success stories can provide those with diabetes encouragement, motivation, and practical insights to help them on their path to better health.

Consult a healthcare provider before making any significant changes to your diet, exercise routine, or supplement regimen, particularly if you are taking medication or have pre-existing health issues. With the support of qualified professionals, self-care, and empowerment, people with diabetes can improve their health and well-being and recover control over their lives and futures.

All The Best

Made in the USA
Las Vegas, NV
24 January 2025

16856974R00059